NATIONAL PHYSIOTHERAPY RESEARCH NETW

Getting involved in research
a pocket guide

Edited by Ann P Moore and Philippa Lyon

Copyright The Chartered Society of Physiotherapy and The National Physiotherapy Research Network © 2009.

National Physiotherapy Research Network - a pocket guide

ISBN: 978-1-904400-26-4

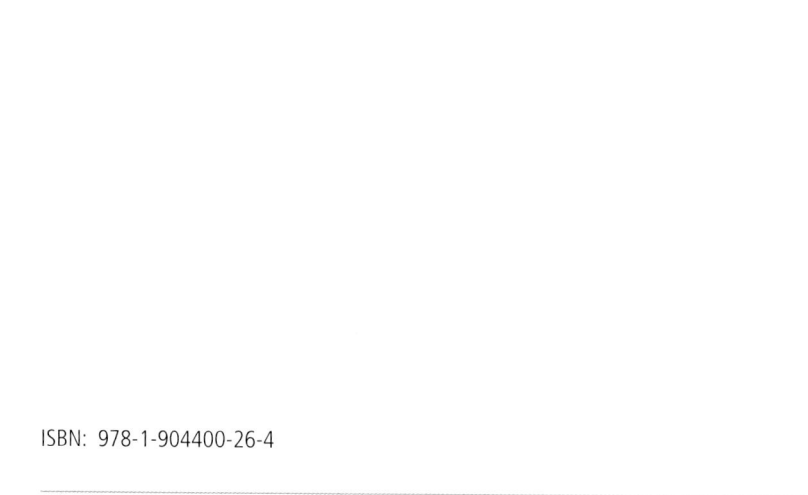

Contents

Foreword – Jill Higgins		**6**
Acknowledgments		**8**
Part One: Engaging in research		
1.1	**Introduction** Ann Moore	**10**
1.2	**How to start** Maria Stokes, Anne Bruton	**14**
1.3	**Searching and appraising the literature** Andrea Peace	**20**
1.4	**Deciding on the right research approach** Graham Stew	**26**
1.5	**Which research methods to use?** Graham Stew	**32**
1.6	**Research ethics and governance** Elizabeth White and Helen Hampson	**40**
1.7	**Collaboration and multidisciplinary research** Gail Mountain	**48**
1.8	**Applying for research funding** Sue Mawson	**54**
1.9	**Collecting good quality data** Anne Bruton and Caroline Ellis-Hill	**60**
1.10	**Analysis of data** Julius Sim	**66**
1.11	**Strategies for dissemination of research** Krysia Dziedzic	**72**
1.12	**Writing for publication** Philippa Lyon	**80**
1.13	**Writing for scientific publications: tips from an editor** Michele Harms	**86**

1.14 **Integrating your own research into practice**   92
Mindy Cairns

1.15 **Using evidence in practice**   100
Bernadette Henderson

1.16 **Creating and sustaining supportive environments for research**   108
Lisa Roberts and Stuart Fraser

1.17 **Mentorship: an overview**   113
Claudia Fellmer

1.18 **Mentorship schemes: an example**   120
Adam Garrow

Part Two: Developing research skills and expertise through education and career pathways

2.1 **Developing a research career pathway**   124
Gabrielle Rankin

2.2 **The new graduate's first steps into research**   133
Suzanne McDonough and David Baxter

2.3 **Registering on a Professional Doctorate programme**   138
Nikki Petty

2.4 **Registering on a traditional PhD programme**   142
Liz Cousins

2.5 **Life after completing a PhD**   151
Brona McDowell

2.6 **The route from novice to Principal Investigator**   156
Di Newham

2.7 **A senior physiotherapist with a postgraduate masters degree: developing research interests**   160
Janet Deane

2.8 **Contract research staff roles**   160
Sally Singh

2.9	**A junior contract researcher** Rupert Kerrell	**164**
2.10	**A clinical researcher** Rhoda Allison	**170**
2.11	**An experienced researcher** Nadine E Foster	**174**
2.12	**A lecturer** Lorna Paul	**180**
2.13	**A researching consultant** Laura Finucane	**186**
2.14	**Leading clinical research** Jeremy Lewis	**192**
2.15	**Research-oriented manager** Fiona Ottewell	**196**

Glossary — **200**

Brief Biographies of Contributors — **210**

Foreword
Dr Jill Higgins Director of Practice and Development
Chartered Society of Physiotherapy

Research and the use of evidence to determine what we do, why and how we do it, is fundamental to the provision of high quality physiotherapy.

Physiotherapy, along with other allied health professions, is well placed to lead high quality evidence-based health and well-being services, and ensure excellence in patient care. However, there are areas where the evidence base for physiotherapy practice is less robust and it was this need to invest in the development of the evidence base, and therefore the capacity for research within the profession, that prompted the Chartered Society of Physiotherapy (CSP) to fund the establishment of the National Physiotherapy Research Network.

It is true to say that the physiotherapy research community and the CSP have not always seen eye to eye, and as in most cases of disagreement, much was the result of each party not understanding the other.

This book is a tangible demonstration of the journey that both the CSP and the physiotherapy research community have taken towards increasingly understanding the needs and demands of the other. In 2004 the CSP took the decision to appoint a team of individuals from four different universities to lead the 'grass root' development of research capacity. Some four years later the National Physiotherapy Research Network is well established, with 20 regional hubs covering the whole of the UK and two hubs in Southern Ireland.

The creation of this book mirrors the commitment and professionalism of all concerned in the development and implementation of the NPRN, who have given substantial time, knowledge and support to enable individuals to engage with research both, as researchers and as users of research. It is testament to the altruistic vision of the NPRN that this book is designed to help develop physiotherapy as a profession as well as develop the individual physiotherapist or other allied health professional.

The book is in two parts. In part one there is straightforward guidance on the various aspects of the research process from how to start and decide on the right approach to ethics and applying for funding. There is a useful section on multidisciplinary research and collaboration – a 'must do' in the current integrated health and well-being environment – plus how to get good quality data and what to do with it. As a profession physiotherapy is not as good as it might be on implementation of the evidence base so part one culminates with sections on publication, dissemination and using research in your own practice.

Part two addresses how to embark upon a career as a researcher and various authors share their personal stories of how the journeys they have made have contributed to the evidence for physiotherapy. This book is different from other research texts, giving as it does personal stories from physiotherapy researchers about how to succeed in research. The book does not profess to give all the answers, but does put research and the development of the evidence base for practice into the 'real world' context of the physiotherapy practitioner. It aims to assist all those already engaged in, or who are thinking about engaging in research, to find the most successful path.

JH

Acknowledgments
Ann Moore and Philippa Lyon

The achievements of the National Physiotherapy Research Network (NPRN) in supporting and encouraging clinicians to engage with research have been made through the expertise, dedication and goodwill of a group of researchers and clinicians. These researchers have freely given their time, knowledge and skills in the interests of developing physiotherapy research capacity in the UK. It is indicative of the loyalty and farsightedness of the physiotherapy profession and other AHPs that a voluntary organisation such as NPRN can be created and sustained. The efforts of those involved in NPRN are made in the interest of producing research that will underpin the evidence base for the future.

We would like to give our warmest thanks and appreciation to all the contributors to this book who have, in the spirit of NPRN, contributed their work out of goodwill. In many cases, these authors have given personal insights and described their own experiences, as well as summarising key points and pieces of advice on their particular topic area. We hope that this shared experience encourages and supports other colleagues to step further into the world of research, and to contribute to the continual strengthening of AHPs as researching professions.

Quotation:
'Research is a high-hat word that scares a lot of people. It needn't... it is nothing but a state of mind, a friendly welcoming attitude to change. It is the problem-solving mind. It is the composer mind instead of the fiddler mind. It is the tomorrow mind instead of the yesterday mind.' (Kettering CF 1961)

1.1 Introduction
Ann Moore

A warm welcome to this tome! It is with great pleasure that on behalf of the National Physiotherapy Research Network (NPRN) Core Executive, I introduce this book which has received voluntary contributions from 40 authors who are all researchers and many of whom are highly experienced researchers, eminent in their fields of practice and/or their research areas.

The NPRN was established in 2004 as a result of a funding initiative by the Chartered Society of Physiotherapy (CSP). The initiative was designed to enhance physiotherapy research capacity and capability in the UK. Four Core Executive members, Di Newham, Julius Sim, Maureen Simmons (now replaced by Maria Stokes) and myself, Ann Moore, put forward a proposal to the CSP to develop a UK-wide network of research hubs to facilitate support and nurture physiotherapy research and the use of evidence in practice. The proposal was successful and the network began its development with the employment of Philippa Lyon as the NPRN Research Officer. We have been delighted with the rapid development of 20 research hubs in England, Northern Ireland, Scotland and Wales, and also the inclusion of two hubs in Southern Ireland. Each of the hubs works within a different model to suit local needs and expertise, and they are all facilitated by an experienced researcher, or a team of experienced researchers. (Please see the Appendix of this handbook for more information relating to the NPRN support hubs, together with useful contact numbers.) Many of the NPRN hubs have gone from strength to strength, holding regular events and meetings which are attended by physiotherapists, but also increasingly by other allied health professionals, and to this end there is a proposal to develop the network further to become the Allied Health Professions Research Network, supporting all allied health professionals interested in research at grass roots level and engendering cooperation and collaboration to fulfill a shared purpose, the development of a sound and accessible evidence base for healthcare practice.

Why is research important and why should any health professional get involved in research? As health professionals we all wish to offer the highest quality of care to our patients, the best quality teaching and learning experiences for our students and present strong coherent information to managers and commissioners of our services. The only way we can fulfil stakeholders' needs is by producing strong and meaningful evidence on which to base our care, our interaction with patients, our service delivery, our cost-effectiveness calculations and our curricula.

Bailey once defined research as 'any activity undertaken to increase knowledge. It is the systematic investigation of a problem, issue or question.' (Bailey DM, 1991) This is a great definition as it really indicates that research can occur at a range of levels, through a range of activities, using a spectrum of approaches and methods.

A characteristic of research is that it challenges the status quo, for example, research findings may indicate that a well known, well used treatment modality is not as effective as everybody thinks. This can be seen as a tremendous challenge for some individuals, but importantly contextual issues are key and just because a treatment modality has been found to be less effective, it doesn't mean that it should necessarily be abandoned. The research needs to be examined closely for rigour and clinical applicability to ascertain if the findings are meaningful for the said situation. The research may indicate that perhaps we need to know more about how a treatment can be best applied, ie in terms of dosage and frequency and perhaps rigour of application, or does it mean that this type of treatment appears to suit patients with particular demographic/clinical profiles? Perhaps the clinical expertise of those delivering the treatment in the study could be challenged and perhaps the outcomes were not measured at appropriate times. So as you can see, research can not only be challenging, but often also leads to a sequence of further questions which can stimulate debate and further research work. Research is also creative, is systematic and fascinating because it enables the researcher to think creatively about how the research could be carried out, using of course recognised frameworks and approaches. It necessitates the researcher to delve deeply into the supporting literature, resulting often in new knowledge for the individual concerned. The research process can trigger new thoughts about how, when and for how long treatment should be applied, what adjuncts to treatment can be used and, who should be involved in the study. In other words who are the real stakeholders in this research?

Research ultimately can lead to changes in what treatments are delivered, how they are delivered, who delivers them, who should receive such treatment and when they should receive it. Research using qualitative methods can also enable us to understand in greater depth our treatment approaches, our examination approaches and, our communication skills from patients' and other stakeholders' perspectives. We can then begin to understand how patients feel about participating in their own self management and what types of treatment and approaches they feel are of benefit and why this is the case. Increasingly, mixed methods approaches are being undertaken, which as well as exploring the effectiveness of treatments from a quantitative perspective, also help us to understand why they were or were not effective from the patient's perspective. But research isn't just about collecting information or data from participants in a systematic way. It can also involve reviewing the literature systematically, the result of which would be a systematic review. Examples of different types of research are given throughout the text.

The book is presented in two sections: Section 1 deals with the research process and each chapter reflects a different stage in this process; Section 2, on the other hand, contains chapters in which researchers at different stages of career development, and having different roles in academic/clinical communities, talk about their experiences of research and their individual growth as researchers. We are indebted to all the contributors to this book who have done so to support the National Physiotherapy Research Network activities. The short biographies of the contributors bear witness to their personal development and growth as researchers and make interesting reading in parallel with their written contributions.

The production of this book is a non profit-making venture for the editors and authors and any profit made from sales will be used to support research activities within the National Physiotherapy Research Network. We do hope you enjoy reading the handbook and reflecting on the content and we hope it may inspire you to play a bigger part in your local research culture, whether you are a student, a clinician, a researcher, a lecturer or a manager.

Some therapists feel demoralised and threatened by their own perceived lack of research skills. If you feel this way you are not alone! But don't be disheartened. We have a large evidence base to construct and really only clinicians know what meaningful research questions need to be answered to support clinical practice. So it is important that all clinicians engage in research at a range of levels, bearing in mind that not every clinician can fully engage in collecting research data. There just isn't time or the resources to do so.

This book was conceived by the Core Executive of the National Physiotherapy Research Network and is designed to whet your appetite in terms of getting involved in research. The chapters are purposely brief and to the point, but written in what we hope is a user-friendly manner. The book is not designed to be a definitive research textbook. There are many texts available on the market today which would fulfil the definitive text remit. A number of these texts are referenced within this handbook. This handbook then is more of a guide to stimulate and hopefully enthuse the would-be research student or the would-be researcher, whether based in clinical practice or in academia. Many of the stand-alone chapters carry useful references, but also reference to further information to deepen knowledge gained. A glossary of terms is provided at the end of the handbook for clarification of perhaps less familiar terms.

Anyone can be involved in research at a number of different levels, whether it is helping to develop a research question, helping with designing research, collecting data, helping with the analysis or the interpretation of the analysis of data, taking part in the dissemination of research, implementing research into clinical practice or incorporating research into teaching and learning experiences. You don't have to be an expert to be involved in research and as your expertise grows you can be involved in more elements of research. The chapters in this book will show you how you can be involved and how research careers and responsibilities are focused. The quotation by Kettering at the beginning of this book couldn't be more apt for this context. So don't be afraid to get involved in research, have courage and let your interest in research flow positively into involvement in research. Why not start today!

Reference
Bailey D. M 1991 Research for the Health Professional – a practical guide. FA Davis Company, Philadelphia

1.2 How to start
Maria Stokes and Anne Bruton

Routes to starting ~ research pathway ~ proposal preparation ~ precautions

Routes to starting

Before starting any activity, it helps to have a reasonably good idea about what you think you want to achieve. This does not mean you cannot change your mind later, but is a good starting point. Research activity is no different. So, firstly you need to ask yourself:

Why do I want to get involved in research?
The answers to this basic question can be many and varied, but the advice in this chapter will relate to the more common reasons:
- There is a clinical problem/question I want to be able to answer.
- I want to work towards a postgraduate qualification (MSc/PhD/DClinP and so on)
- I enjoyed the research I did while training and would like to do some more, but do not have sufficient time or confidence to develop independent research
- I did not gain any practical experience of research while training but like the idea of getting involved.

You may have other, more personal, reasons: for example you think it will help you get promotion; you like the idea of seeing your name in print; you want to move into a research career – it really doesn't matter – what matters is that you get started. After a while, we hope you will want to do research because you discover it is productive, challenging and exciting.

The first thing to realise is that you cannot start out in research on your own. Whom you contact first may vary depending on your research requirements. So, for the situations mentioned above:
- If you want to answer a particular clinical question, you need to find a mentor who has sufficient research experience to guide you through the process. Depending on where you work, this may be a physiotherapy (or other health professional) colleague, or a local academic.
- If you want to work towards a higher degree or other postgraduate qualification, you need to check out university websites or contact university departments.
- If you want to do research but do not have sufficient time or skills for a complete project, you could think about getting involved with research projects that are already up and running. To find out about these, you could contact your local Research Support Unit (RSU)/Research Design Service (RDS) or National

FIGURE 1

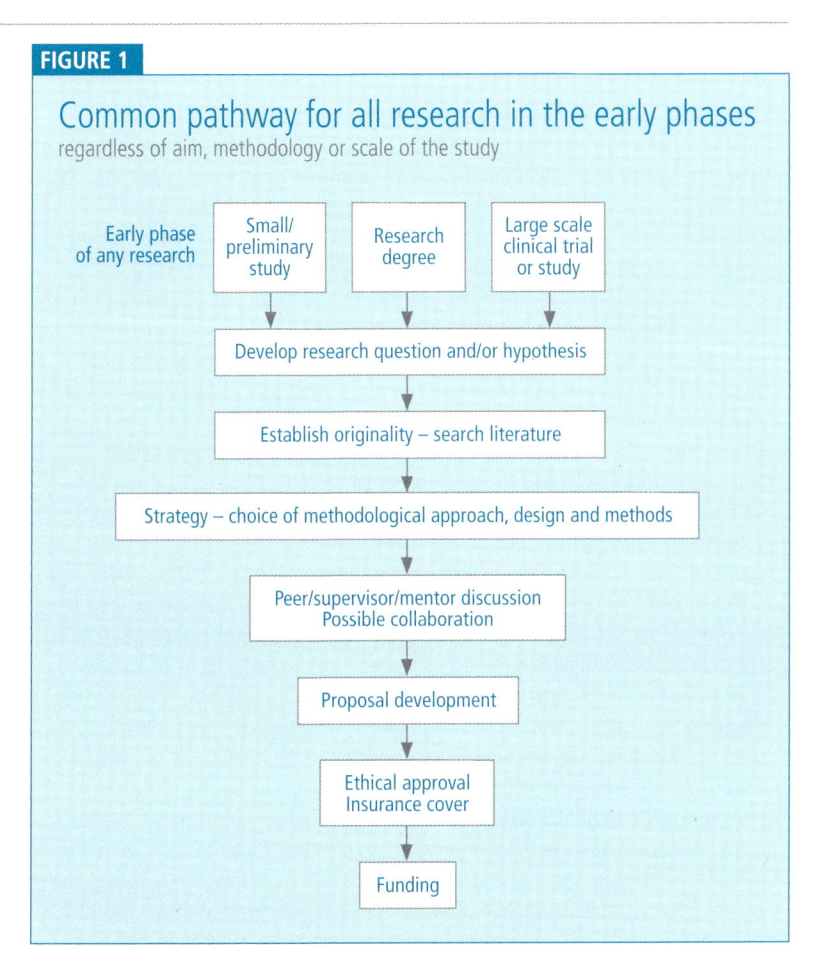

Common pathway for all research in the early phases
regardless of aim, methodology or scale of the study

```
                    ┌──────────────┐   ┌──────────┐   ┌──────────────┐
                    │   Small/     │   │          │   │  Large scale │
  Early phase       │ preliminary  │   │ Research │   │ clinical trial│
  of any research   │   study      │   │  degree  │   │   or study   │
                    └──────┬───────┘   └────┬─────┘   └──────┬───────┘
                           ▼                ▼                ▼
                    Develop research question and/or hypothesis
                                        ▼
                    Establish originality – search literature
                                        ▼
           Strategy – choice of methodological approach, design and methods
                                        ▼
                    Peer/supervisor/mentor discussion
                         Possible collaboration
                                        ▼
                            Proposal development
                                        ▼
                             Ethical approval
                             Insurance cover
                                        ▼
                                   Funding
```

Physiotherapy Research Network (NPRN) hub, consult the National Research Register (NRR; website address listed in further information) or look at the website of your local university to find out what is going on in your geographical area. Think about what skills you might have to offer an existing project; perhaps clinical skills, assisting with literature searching, analysing results. Also be clear about what you can reasonably expect from your involvement, such as being a named author or included in the acknowledgments of a paper. This needs to be negotiated appropriately before you begin any actual involvement.

Common pathway
All research has a common pathway in the early phases (see Figure 1):
- **Research question and/or hypothesis:** The first (and sometimes the most difficult) step is to define the question/s that you hope to answer as precisely as possible. This may appear to be a fairly straightforward process but it can take several weeks to refine your initial question. Example: you might start off by asking 'Does breathing retraining help people with asthma?' After much thinking and discussion you might expand your question to make it more specific, such as: 'How does four weeks of daily Papworth breathing retraining affect health-related quality of life and symptom control in people with mild to moderate asthma, compared with daily exercise on a cycle ergometer?' You would then refine it further and further until you end up with your final version, but try to keep it simple and clear.
- **Originality:** You need to establish if this question has been posed/answered before. It is not ethical to do research if the answer is already known and has been demonstrated conclusively. This is fairly rare in physiotherapy research. Repeating studies to confirm previous findings (for example in a different setting) is usually acceptable. This is where a thorough literature search is essential. If the question has not been addressed at all, then either you have an amazingly novel idea or there is a reason no one has tried (for example too difficult; unethical; too expensive). More commonly you find some people have answered a piece of your question but not enough to give clinical certainty.
- **Strategy:** You need to work out how to answer your research question that is what method to use. The choice of qualitative or quantitative methods, or mixed methodology, will depend on the question posed.
- **Peer discussion/collaboration:** Start to share your ideas with friends/colleagues/mentor/supervisor and get as much feedback as possible. Try not to take their criticisms personally – they are trying to help you. Explore possible collaboration with relevant colleagues in your own or other disciplines. Collaborative research is likely to be more productive than single investigator efforts, particularly if you collaborate with more experienced researchers than yourself.
- **Resources:** Work out how long you think the research will take and how much it will cost – can you find the time and money within your own department/private practice, or do you need to seek external funding? There is very little scope for unfunded research in the health service. Do you need a research assistant to collect the data? Statistical support may be necessary to help with the study design, and plans for data management and statistical analysis. Access to statistical support requires good planning and needs to be arranged at an early stage. It may be too late to go to a

statistician with data, as they may not have been collected appropriately for being processed and presented in a meaningful way.

Work out a timetable for the project and remember it is not just for the data collection period. You also need to allow time for:
- **Literature review:** ongoing throughout, not just at the beginning.
- **Preparing paperwork/databases** for data collection.
- **Research governance** (website address listed below): formal peer review of your protocol, submitting for ethical approval, waiting for ethical approval, insurance cover and so on.
- **Recruitment:** it is an unwritten law that as soon as you start to study something, the whole population with that problem seems to disappear – always expect recruitment to be much slower than you originally anticipated.
- **Delays:** absence through illness/annual leave may affect you or others on whom progress of the study depends.
- **Post-data collection:** data analysis and writing up.
- **Proposal preparation:** see next section.
- **Funding:** see chapter 1.8.

Proposal preparation

A research proposal is essentially a statement of intent – the plan or roadmap to inform yourself and others (ethics committees, R&D departments, potential funders and so on) about what you are going to do. Before writing the proposal, find out the submission deadlines for your local ethics committee and whether the proposal must first be approved by your Head of Department and/or institution before submission.

Once the details of the protocol in your proposal are finalised you are committed to following them precisely – any deviation is a very serious matter as it renders you liable to losing your insurance and indemnity cover, the study being halted and results not being publishable. This is why it is so important to get it right before you start. If you wish to make changes to your protocol, you may only do so by requesting approval for amendments from the ethics committee (and research governance office for insurance cover) and waiting for written approval before you change anything. It is advisable to familiarise yourself with research governance requirements which aim to ensure that health and social care research is conducted to high scientific and ethical standards (see website address below). Research proposals generally follow a common format with the headings in Box 1 and useful references include: Portney & Watkins (2000), Sim and Wright (2000).

BOX 1
Writing a research proposal

- Title – reflects what you are planning to do
- Summary/abstract – brief outline of the study
- Lay description: brief outline of the study in language that an adult with a reading age of 14 years or above would understand
- Background/introduction – 'set the scene' that is introduce the topic and why it needs to be studied. Give a brief literature review of relevant previous work and highlight the gap in knowledge that your research will fill
- Aims/objectives/hypotheses – aims are essentially the 'big' research question/s. Objectives are the steps you need to take to achieve the overall aim. Some quantitative research lends itself to forming hypotheses – statements that are testable (usually statistically)
- Significance – state relevance of the study to the subject population and/or health services in general and/or scientific knowledge. May include: improvements in care/treatment; benefit to health and/or quality of life; market potential
- Methods – subject population, inclusion/exclusion criteria, sample size, how you will recruit; research design (type of study for example experimental, qualitative); equipment/instrumentation; protocol that is data collection process from recruitment to completion; data analysis plans; dissemination of findings
- Ethical considerations – how subjects will be recruited, discomfort to subjects, known side effects of treatment and how these will be minimised, any inconvenience to patients/relatives and so on
- Governance issues – for example taking up NHS staff time, disruption to ward routine
- Time scale – see above. Use a flow chart if possible
- Brief CV of investigators – usually one page – qualifications, previous and present positions, membership of scientific societies, research funding, number of publications
- Costs – staff, equipment, travel and so on
- References to the literature.

In addition to the protocol, ethics committees will also expect there to be appendices, including examples of any questionnaires, data collection forms, consent forms, participant information sheets, recruitment letters/posters/emails.

Precautions

Most people involved in research are ethical and honest. However, if you have some good new research ideas you may need to be cautious about how freely you share them. Intellectual property (often shortened to IP) is a term to describe your original ideas and this IP is owned by your institution, as part of research governance (see further information). You need to protect your IP in the same way that you might protect any other valuable possessions. If all you want is to get your research question answered, then this may not worry you. However, if you want to try to obtain funding and then publish your findings – it is exasperating to find someone else has taken your ideas and done so first. After initial discussion of an idea in principle, a Confidentiality Agreement is often drawn up between parties and if the idea develops into a project, a Collaboration Agreement may be signed. Protection of IP is most important for ideas with commercial potential and advice can be sought from your local research governance office, usually based in the RSU/RDS.

Networks
First steps are always hard but the hardest part is making the decision that you will start. Trying to go it alone is not advisable and you are likely to give up very quickly. Those of us experienced in research know how much we depend on each other. There are formal networks like the NPRN ready to help you and there are informal networks that you can help create within your own department/area. Academic researchers are not failed clinicians living in ivory towers but are useful resources who can work with you to help you achieve what you want. Although there are one or two sharks in the pool of academia, there are many more dolphins around who genuinely want to help increase research capacity within the allied health professions.

Reference list
- Portney LG, Watkins MP. Editors (2000) Foundations of Clinical Research: Applications to Practice. 2nd edn. Prentice-Hall Health. London.
- Sim J, Wright C. (2000) Research in Health Care: Concepts, Designs and Methods. Stanley Thornes Ltd. Cheltenham.

Further information
National Research Register: **www.nrr.nhs.uk**
Research governance Framework for Health and Social Care: **www.dh.gov.uk/en/ Policyandguidance/Researchanddevelopment/A-Z/Researchgovernance/DH_4002112**
Ethical Issues: **www.nres.npsa.nhs.uk**
Ethics Application Forms: **www.myresearchproject.org.uk**

1.3 Searching and appraising the literature
Andrea Peace

Searching the literature ~ appraising the literature ~ time management ~ reference list ~ further information

Searching the literature

- Why search the literature?
- Defining your research question
- The need for a search strategy
- Sources to search
- Saving/organising your search results
- Documenting/reusing your search strategy
- Support with the literature searching process

Why search the literature?
There are many reasons why you should conduct a literature search including:
- To scope the quantity of published literature on the subject you are interested in researching.
- To locate relevant background reading to help you focus your thinking, and ultimately your research question.
- To reveal identical research to your proposed study, thereby preventing you 'reinventing the wheel'.
- To identify high quality journal articles that will inform your research.
- To discover similar research to highlight potential future research partners.

Defining your research question
The PICO system (Richardson et al, 1995) is an evidence-based model for creating clinical research questions. It encourages the researcher to break down a clinical scenario into a question which can be answered typically through a combination of reviewing the relevant literature, and undertaking some original research.

A research scenario could be elderly men experiencing falls; should this be treated through exercise classes or individual home visits? This could be broken down, using the PICO system, into the following elements:
- the patient or population (who?)
  – elderly men.
- the intervention (what?)
  – exercise classes.

- the comparison (optional)
  - home visits.
- the outcome (how is it measured?)
  - reduced incidence of falls.

The ECLIPSE system (Wildridge and Bell, 2002) is a tool to help break down health management/policy scenarios into concepts, which can form the basis of your search:
- **Expectation**
  - Reduction of waiting times in a musculoskeletal physiotherapy outpatient service.
- **Client group**
  - People with musculoskeletal injuries.
- **Location**
  - Hospital outpatients.
- **Impact**
  - Reduced waiting times; increased patient satisfaction; increased job satisfaction; increased efficiency.
- **Professionals**
  - Physiotherapists.
- **Service**
  - Musculoskeletal physiotherapy outpatients.

In both the PICO and ECLIPSE models, the individual elements of the broken-down scenario form the building blocks of your literature search.

The need for a search strategy

Bearing in mind that there is an enormous body of published literature in the medical/health field, you need to formulate a search strategy to ensure you retrieve only literature that is relevant to your research question.

Questions to consider when drawing up the strategy:
- What question are you trying to answer?
- Using a model like PICO or ECLIPSE what individual elements make up this question?
  - you need to use these to identify a list of keywords to search in combination to retrieve the relevant literature.
- Are alternative terms and spellings relevant? for example physical therapy; physiotherapy.
- Is date of publication relevant? – by using a publication date limit, your search will capture literature published within your specified timeframe.
- Is the scope of the research context specific (for example UK health system)?

1.3

- consider using a 'place of publication' limit within your search.
- Is language important? – for example if you can only read English or there is no funding available for translating articles then consider applying an 'English only' language limitation within your search.
- Is research methodology important? – for example you want to retrieve only randomised control trials or systematic reviews, and not individual case studies, then consider excluding certain types of methodology from your search.

Individual bibliographic databases vary considerably in terms of how they allow the user to input the search strategy (that is how you can combine your keywords and apply limits). Investing some time in reading the online help facility before conducting a search of an individual database or library catalogue is critical to ensure you retrieve only relevant references.

Sources to search

The next step is to choose appropriate sources to search for relevant published literature. The sources chosen will vary depending on the subject in question. General health bibliographic databases like Medline, CINAHL or the Cochrane Library tackle a wide range of subjects, whereas databases like Pedro, or OTSeeker bring together research from one discipline (in this case physiotherapy, and occupational therapy respectively).

Library catalogues also provide a useful resource particularly in locating books and reports on the subject in question. Finally, the internet is a good place to search for government reports, statistics, and reports from other healthcare research organisations. However, internet search engines are generally a poor alternative to bibliographic databases when searching for high quality research.

Saving/organising your search results

Most bibliographic databases allow you to mark references of interest to save, email or print. When undertaking research that will result in an extensive reference list, it is good practice to save the references within a personal bibliographic software package (for example Endnote, Reference Manager or Procite). These packages allow you to sort and format references in a particular referencing style (for example Vancouver, Harvard). They can integrate with your word-processing software to insert references within the text, and compile an automatic bibliography saving valuable time in the publishing process.

Documenting/reusing your search strategy

Most bibliographic databases provide an option to save (and rerun) search strategies.

This feature records the combination of terms and limits you used to run your search. This is useful as you may be required to publish your search strategy as part of your research findings. Also, using your saved search strategy you can run repeat searches at specified intervals to collect newly published literature on your research question in a consistent manner.

Support with the literature searching process
Developing skills takes time and effort, but improves with practice; this is the same with literature searching. If you are struggling, ask a librarian to review your draft search strategy. They should be able to point out any omissions, suggest alternative keywords, recommend and train you to search appropriate bibliographic databases, and advise on downloading, storing and manipulating records in a personal bibliographic software package.

Appraising the literature

- Why appraise the literature?
- The advantages of using critical appraisal in the research process
- Tools to carry out critical appraisal

Why appraise the literature?
Once the literature search is complete, it is important to examine the quality and validity of the information located. 'Critical appraisal' is the process of systematically assessing research evidence to decide on the relative quality of the results and recommendations. Depending on the outcome of each critical appraisal, you will either include or exclude each article from your literature review based on whether you feel the article is good enough to help inform your research.

The advantages of using critical appraisal in the research process
The advantages are that it:
- provides an objective assessment of the usefulness of individual pieces of research
- helps you to manage information overload by eliminating certain studies from being considered in your research
- aids decision making regarding whether to take published research evidence and put it into practice.

1.3

Tools to carry out critical appraisal

There has been much investment in creating free critical appraisal tools; these usually take the form of a standardised questionnaire, which lead you to reflect on different aspects of the research (for example research design, bias and so on).

Different tools exist to critically appraise articles that use different types of research methodology. You need to identify the type of research described in the article you want to review (for example systematic review), and then search for a systematic review critical appraisal tool.

The following free resources are available to help aid your critical appraisal:

AGREE instrument (appraisal tool for assessing clinical guidelines):
http://www.agreecollaboration.org/pdf/agreeinstrumentfinal.pdf

Critical Appraisal Skills Programme – Appraisal Tools (includes tools to review: systematic reviews; randomised controlled trials; economic evaluation studies; cohort studies; qualitative research; case control studies; diagnostic test studies):
http://www.phru.nhs.uk/Pages/PHD/resources.htm

Time management

Searching and appraising the literature can be time consuming. Not only is there a search strategy to develop and run in a variety of sources, time also needs to be built in for ordering your selected references (this may take several weeks if they have to come from other libraries). Time also needs to be allocated to critically appraising your selected references, so give enough time to each of these steps in your research project plan. However this time is an investment, and your research should reap the benefits by considering only relevant and high quality research in its considerations.

Reference list

Richardson WS, Wilson MC, Nishikawa J, Hayward RS. (1995) The well-built clinical question: a key to evidence-based decisions. ACP Journal Club 123: A12-A13.
Wildridge V, Bell L. (2002) How CLIP became ECLIPSE: a mnemonic to assist in searching for health policy/management information. Health Information and Libraries Journal 19: 113-115.

Further information

Searching:
- The Chartered Society of Physiotherapy. (2007) CSP guide to literature searching, 3rd edition. The Chartered Society of Physiotherapy, London. Please note – this is a CSP member only publication available via the CSP website **http://www.csp.org.uk**
- National Library for Health Knowledge Management Specialist Library (n.d.). Search strategy used to find content for the Knowledge Management Specialist Library. **http://www.library.nhs.uk/SpecialistLibrarysearch/Download. aspx?resID=101412**. An example of a PICO saved search strategy that has been run on a bibliographic database.
- South Central Healthcare Librarians. (2007) The Literature Search Process: Protocols for Researchers, 2nd edition. Thames Valley Health Libraries Network, Thames Valley. **http://www.library.nhs.uk/knowledgemanagement/Page. aspx?pagename=RZHOME**

Appraising:
- Booth A, Brice A (2004) Appraising the evidence. In: Booth A, Brice A (eds) Evidence-based practice for Information Professionals. Facet Publishing, London, 104-119. **http://www.facetpublishing.co.uk/481.pdf**
- University of Sheffield School of Health and Related Research (n.d.). Critical appraisal and using the literature, Sheffield. **http://www.shef.ac.uk/scharr/ir/units/critapp/ index.htm**
An online tutorial covering the basics of critical appraisal.

1.4 Deciding on the right research approach
Graham Stew

Research paradigms ~ methodologies ~ conclusions ~ recommended reading

Having selected your research question (see 1.2), and identified what your aims are (that is what you want your research to produce as an outcome), the next issue is to think about the best approach for your study. In other words, what design or general strategy will be the most appropriate for finding the answers to your research question? These strategies are also known as *methodologies*.

- How do you find the best methodology?
- Start with your research question!

What are you asking? The wording of your question will usually indicate what the answers will look like.

> Research can do several things, depending on the type of question asked. It can:
> - Describe
> - Interpret
> - Explain
> - Predict
> - Offer some evidence
> - Evaluate

Knowing what you want your research to do helps you to identify the correct approach. If little is known about your research topic, and it has not been researched much, if at all, then you might need to describe, interpret or explain. This type of reasoning, from the particular to the general, is known as induction.

As our knowledge of a subject increases we are able to predict relationships between the variables in our study, and make an educated guess as to the outcome of our research – an hypothesis. So if the knowledge base is already established and you are building upon previous studies, your research may well need to predict, offer some evidence or evaluate. This reasoning, from the general to the particular, is known as deduction.

Our understanding of any subject requires both inductive and deductive reasoning, as each is needed to complement the other at different stages of knowledge development.

Research paradigms

A paradigm is simply a way of looking at the world... a theoretical lens or perspective. Working within a research paradigm means having certain ideas of what reality (ontology) and knowledge (epistemology) mean.

This is not the place to go deeply into these issues, but all researchers need to ask themselves where they stand in relation to these philosophical questions. For example, do you believe that we create our own realities through interpreting our experience, and that knowledge is therefore subjective and relative? Or do you feel that the world exists independently of the observer, and that knowledge is 'out there', waiting to be discovered?

Broadly speaking, the first position falls within the interpretivist paradigm, while the second would be within a positivist paradigm.

Both paradigms may use common methods of data collection (that is questionnaires), and the data may be both qualitative and quantitative in any research study.

There needs to be a comfortable 'fit' between the paradigm and research question adopted; between the researcher's worldview and the type of reasoning to be used.

But enough of philosophy!... let's consider some practical examples of research studies.

Methodologies

Within each research paradigm there is a wide and bewildering array of methodologies, but we will focus on six common designs in this chapter.

Let's take low back pain as an example of a research topic to illustrate these methodologies. It's a subject that is relevant to therapists everywhere, and you might think that a sound body of knowledge already exists on this subject. However it could be equally argued that an individual's experience of, and response to, back pain is unique and non-generalisable. Everything depends on the question you are asking as a researcher (... and of course your paradigm!).

1.4

Here are six specific methodologies, related to different research questions, and the six purposes of research:

- **Survey**
Research seeking to describe may ask:
'What is the prevalence of low back pain among retired nurses?'

A survey design is a specific approach to collecting social data. It involves collecting the same data from cases in a sample, and may use questionnaires, structured interviews, telephone interviews and medical records.

- **Phenomenology**
Research that describes and interprets will ask patients:
'Can you tell me about your experience of back pain?'

Phenomenology as a research methodology seeks to describe the lived experience of individuals, with a view to increasing our understanding of a phenomenon. Hermeneutic phenomenology also interprets the patients' accounts, developing themes or essences to present shared meanings. Data are normally collected through in-depth individual interviews and sometimes participants' diaries.

- **Grounded Theory**
Research that seeks to create a theory which answers the question:
'What coping strategies do back pain patients adopt?'

Grounded theory seeks to develop a model or theory to explain a social process, in this case, how back pain patients cope with their problem. Data are collected through a range of methods which might include focus group and individual interviews, questionnaires and documentary analysis. Analysis of data proceeds through a process of constant comparison, generating categories which form a conceptual framework or 'substantive' theory.

- **Correlational study**
Research which seeks to predict may ask:
'Is there a correlation between certain symptoms of low back pain and Body Mass Index?'

A correlational study is a systematic investigation of relationships between two or more variables within the research topic, and does not seek to examine cause and effect. Data from the variables are collected and compared to detect significant statistical relationships.

- **Randomised controlled trials**

Research seeking to test an hypothesis might ask:
'Does technique A produce better outcome measures in low back pain patients than technique B?'

Randomised controlled trials (RCTs) are often accepted as the gold standard for comparing different therapeutic modalities. The random allocation of patients avoids a selection bias and clear inclusion and exclusion criteria maintain the focus of the study. The credibility of results is further enhanced by using independent investigators, blinding techniques and validated research tools for data collection.

- **Action research**

Research which seeks to evaluate, implement and develop healthcare services might ask:
'How can services for low back pain patients be improved?'

Action research aims to improve practice, through a longitudinal study of implementation and evaluation of changes, often within a collaborative team approach. Data are collected throughout the process by methods such as interviews, observation and questionnaire.

Conclusion

As you can see the actual methods for collecting data are common across a wide range of research methodologies, and both qualitative and quantitative data can be used in one study to complement each other and strengthen the findings.

It is easy to become confused and overwhelmed by the variety of methodologies you will find in research textbooks. The simple solution is to be guided by your research question and aims. Remind yourself repeatedly of what you are trying to find out, what you are aiming to achieve, and what your answers are likely to look like. This will (i) keep you on track to accomplish your aims, (ii) help you choose the appropriate methodology and methods for collecting and analysing your data, and (iii) guide you in presenting your findings.

1.4

Choosing the right approach in research is like finding the right tools to do the job... everything else falls into place, and the rest is easy!

Further information
- Clough P, Nutbrown C. (2007) A Student's Guide to Methodology. 2nd Edn. Sage, London.
- Creswell JW. (2007) Qualitative Inquiry and Research Design. 2nd Edn. Sage, London.
- Crotty M. (2004) The Foundations of Social Research. Sage, London.
- O'Leary Z. (2005) Researching Real-World Problems Sage, London.
- Phelps R, Fisher K, & Ellis A. (2007) Organising and Managing your Research: A practical guide for Postgraduates. Sage, London.
- Potter S (ed). (2006) Doing Postgraduate Research. 2nd. Edn. Sage, London.

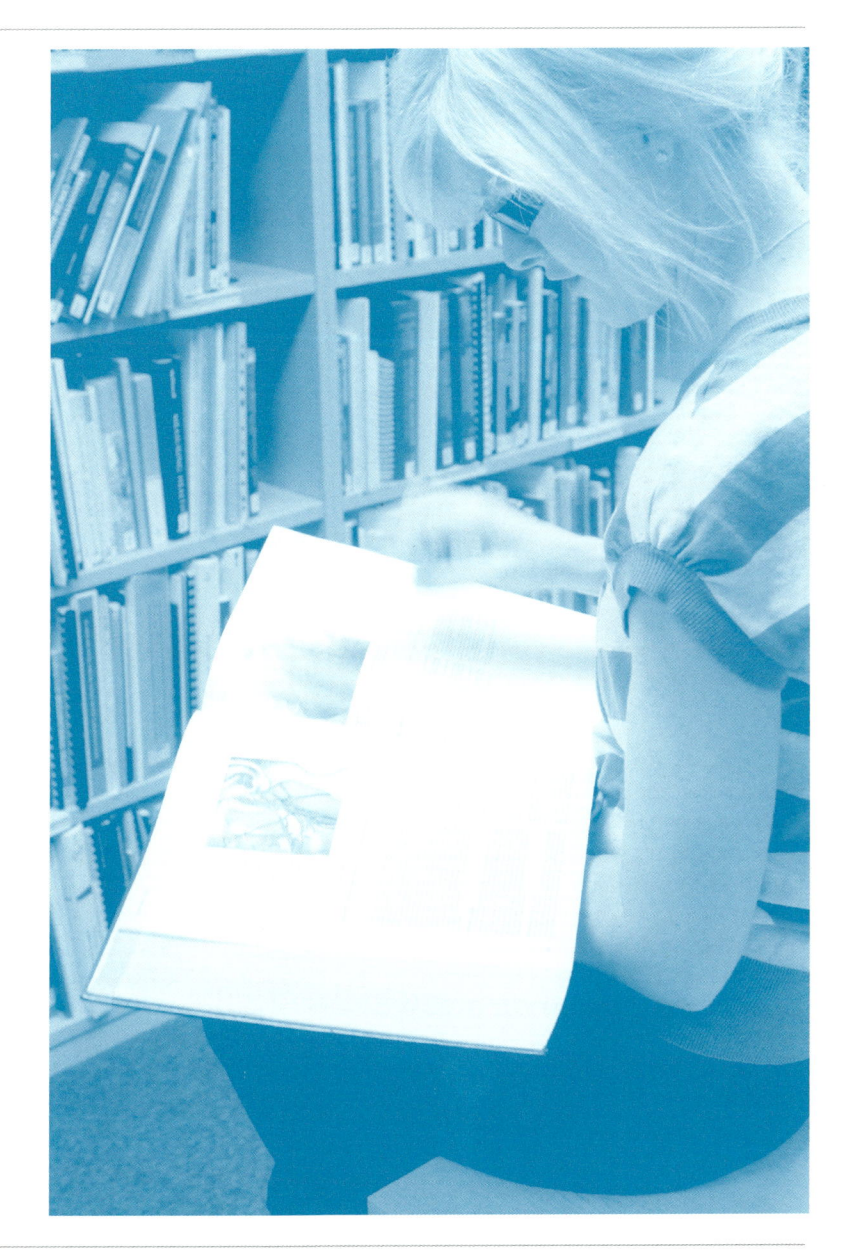

1.5 Which research methods to use?
Graham Stew

Revisit your research question ~ questionnaires ~ interviews ~ focus groups ~ observation ~ documentary analysis ~experiments ~ conclusion

Once you have developed your research question and chosen the appropriate methodology, or overall design, you will now want to consider how to collect the information (the data) you need. These techniques for collecting data will be your research methods.

First, revisit your research question!

A clear question will indicate the type of information you need to answer it.

> Then ask yourself :
> - Where can I find this information?
> - Will this information come from people, equipment, documents, and so on?
> - If from people, who specifically?
> - When can I collect this information?
> - How is this information to be collected and stored?
> - Finally, what methods of analysis will be used?

The first four questions above relate to issues of access and sampling. Access involves knowing where the information is, and how to negotiate your way into the 'field'. If you are researching your own practice and workplace, then access is usually straightforward, but otherwise you will need to know who to approach for approval (the so-called 'gatekeepers'). You will also need to know when and for how long you plan to collect your data. Sampling requires decisions about who has the information you need, and may involve either probability or purposive sampling (see glossary).

The fifth bullet point above refers to the choice of methods of data collection. Both qualitative and quantitative data (words and numbers) may be collected within any research paradigm or design; they can complement each other and in many cases strengthen a piece of research.

> There are many methods of data collection, and this chapter can only address the most common ones, which are:
> - Questionnaires
> - Interviews
> - Focus groups
> - Observation
> - Documentary analysis
> - Experiments

Let's take each in turn, define them, and comment on their advantages and disadvantages:

Questionnaires

These include measurement scales and can be posted to your respondents, sent by email, or administered face-to-face. Questionnaires may be:
- wholly closed-ended, with every question having a fixed range of alternative responses, or;
- open-ended, with very broad questions designed to elicit the respondents' own views rather than their responses to a pre-specified range of answers, or;
- a mixture of the two.

Potential advantages
- Questionnaires are a useful means of getting data from a relatively large number of people or from a representative sample of that population. Therefore they are very efficient in terms of your use of time and effort.
- Respondents may feel that they can say what they really think if the questionnaire can be completed in privacy and anonymously (especially if you are known to them or might be thought to have a vested interest in their answers).
- Questionnaires are also, usually, quicker to code and analyse than interviews.

Potential disadvantages
- Questionnaires may be a quicker method of collecting data and the format may facilitate data analysis, but the design of a good questionnaire with clear instructions and unambiguous questions can take a long time.

1.5

- You may not always know that your carefully constructed questionnaire is not asking the 'right' questions until you start analysing the data, i.e. when it is too late to do anything about it. Pilot your questionnaire if you can. At the very least send it to some colleagues for comment.
- There is a risk that few completed questionnaires are returned – a low response rate is common.
- Respondents may think there is one correct answer and try to find out what this might be – sometimes there is a sense of trying to please the researcher.

Interviews

These are 'conversations with a purpose' (usually face-to-face or by telephone) which are planned around a set of questions or themes. The degree to which interviews are structured can vary greatly. They can be highly structured (and then resemble a verbal questionnaire). They might be semi-structured, comprising a set of open-ended questions but often with follow-up probes and prompts; or they can be relatively unstructured – a list of themes or topics or headings which can be adjusted to each interviewee.

Potential advantages
- Provides an opportunity for the interviewee to give a more detailed response than in a questionnaire.
- The data will usually be richer with more contextual information than the data provided by a questionnaire.
- An interview is a particularly useful tool if you are trying to understand the experiences and actions of each respondent.
- It provides an opportunity to probe respondents' views in ways that might be difficult to plan for in advance.

Potential disadvantages
- The interview is a time-consuming method if you do not have any help in collecting data from a relatively large sample of respondents.
- The full transcription of interviews takes a lot of time. A one-hour tape-recorded interview takes about 8–10 hours to transcribe.
- Good interviewing requires expertise and experience. It requires, for example, good listening skills; body language that encourages the interviewee to relax and talk; a capacity to ask useful questions, perhaps take notes and yet maintain eye contact;

an ability to prompt people who are not very responsive; knowing just how long to allow a silence to continue before intervening; an ability to probe sensitive areas and issues; being able to 'think on your feet' and be flexible in your questioning.

Focus groups

Originally used in market research, this method is now often used in healthcare research. Designed to elicit opinions and attitudes from groups of 6-10 people, focus groups tend to be used in conjunction with other research methods.

Potential advantages
- A cost-effective technique for exploring a group's views without imposing your own agenda on them too strongly.
- Provides opportunities to explore the thinking behind the kinds of responses which might have been given to a questionnaire, without opting for the more time-consuming option of one-to-one interviews.
- In the early stages of a project it can be a useful means of identifying issues or areas of interest that could be followed up using other methods.

Potential disadvantages
- Difficult to follow-up the views of individuals during the group discussion, especially on topics which may be sensitive.
- There may be a need to explore individual experiences more deeply following the focus group. (If it was possible why not opt for face-to-face interviews in the first place?)
- This method can be heavily influenced by the dynamics of the group. One or two people can easily dominate the proceedings if they have clear views and are articulate; others may feel inhibited. It is possible as a facilitator to counter this tendency but it takes experience and self-confidence.
- It may be difficult to tease out what is being said when more than one person speaks at any one time.

Observation

This is the systematic description of events and behaviours in their natural social setting. Observation can be highly structured (with coding schemes, checklists and category systems), or relatively unstructured (taking notes or keeping a diary). As an observer you may be participating in the activities, or be a detached 'fly on the wall'. Crucial to the success of observation as a method is knowing exactly what it is you need to observe, and how to record these data.

Potential advantages
- It is one of the most direct research techniques. You are not asking people what they would do or think; you are watching what they do and listening to what they say.
- Used in combination with questionnaires or interviews, observation can therefore provide useful insights into the extent to which there is a correspondence or discrepancy between what people say and what they actually do.

Potential disadvantages
- It is easy to underestimate the effect of your presence on the situation and behaviour being observed, and gaining informed consent can be a challenge with large numbers of people.
- It is very time consuming… how many times do you need to observe a situation or a group before you can describe with confidence what is really happening?
- The analysis of observational data can be difficult and often open to very different interpretations.

Documentary analysis

You can make use of a wide range of documents related to your research question, including clinical records, minutes of meetings, memoranda, letters, diaries, administrative records; and so on.

Potential advantages
- Documents enable you to investigate the background and context of the situation and the specific problem which interests you.
- Documentary analysis is a useful means of analysing the 'official' view and accessing the 'official' record of events, decisions and plans.
- A useful means of evaluating the extent to which the rhetoric (or the policy) is actually put into practice.

Potential disadvantages
- Documentary analysis, if it is to be systematic, can be time consuming.

- There is little guidance available from experienced researchers on how to analyse some kinds of documents.
- Documents require a critical reading similar to the skills employed by the historian when analysing primary sources. Documents have to be interpreted as well as read and this calls for expertise and experience.

Experiments

The key feature of any experiment is that the researcher controls and manipulates the conditions under which the effects of a change or intervention can be measured. Cohen et al (2000:211) provide a useful brief description of experimental method in the natural sciences:

'Imagine that we have been transported to a laboratory to investigate the properties of a new wonder fertiliser that farmers could use on their cereal crops, let us say wheat. The scientist would take the bag of wheat seed and randomly split it into two equal parts. One part would be the grain under normal existing conditions – controlled and measured amounts of soil, warmth, water and light and no other factors. This would be called the control group. The other part would be grown under the same conditions – the same controlled and measured amounts of soil, warmth and light as the control group but, additionally, the new wonder fertiliser. Then, four months later, the two groups are examined and their growth measured. The control group has grown half a metre and each ear of wheat is in place but the seeds are small. The experimental group, by contrast has grown half a metre as well but has significantly more seeds on each ear, the seeds are larger, fuller and more robust.'

The key features of the experiment are:
- An experimental group and a control group.
- Random allocation to each group to eliminate the possibility that any variables not thought to be crucial to the experiment might have any unintended effects.
- Identification of key variables that will have some effect.
- Control of these key variables.
- The application of the special treatment to the experimental group but not the control group.
- Measurement of the effect of the treatment and comparison of the outcomes for the two groups.

Will this classical experimental design still work when the subjects of the experiment are people rather than wheat seeds?

1.5

The experiment is still the norm in medical research and is widely used in all forms of psychology, research into healthcare and, to a lesser extent, research into social care. One particular form of the experimental design, the randomised controlled trial (through which, for instance, new drugs and forms of medical treatment are tested) is still generally regarded in those disciplines as the 'gold standard' of research.

In each case the experiment is designed in such a way that it reduces the likelihood that the prior knowledge of the subjects, the practitioners and the researchers taking part in the trial might unduly influence the results of the experiment.

However, in many social situations it is simply not practical (or sensible) to try to control all of the possible variables that might influence the outcomes of a specific change or intervention. Indeed, in some instances it would also be unethical to use a controlled experiment if, for instance, the subjects were not in a position to give their informed consent to participation in the experiment or if participation meant that they might suffer or be treated unfairly or if the experiment required them to do something illegal or immoral. Also, in the real world, it may not be possible to assign people randomly to either the experimental or the control group.

In such circumstances some researchers have introduced the idea of a quasi-experiment. Perhaps the most common kinds of quasi-experiment employed in social research are where the researchers collect data that enable them to compare the same subjects before and after an intervention or change has been introduced.

Therefore the quasi-experiment retains the element of comparison which is so central to the experimental research design but subjects are seldom allocated to their groups and, if they are, this is rarely done randomly. In practice, in most quasi-experiments the researcher does not have any control at all over the so-called 'control group' (or reference or comparator group).

Ultimately the central question for any researcher opting for a quasi-experimental design will be: 'Am I comparing like with like?' If the answer is: 'I believe so' then the follow-up question will inevitably be: 'How do I know?'. Also, it is easy to underestimate the amount of time and resources that experimental methods require! There are a variety of different kinds of quasi-experimental research design and each has its own advantages and disadvantages. Rather than outline all of them here it is recommended that you read chapter 4 in Robson (1993).

Additionally, if you are interested in the relative advantages and disadvantages of experimental and quasi-experimental designs for research in healthcare, see Chapter 3 in Gomm & Davies (2000).

Conclusion

This chapter has introduced you to a number of common research methods ... it's now up to you to decide which of them will be of use in answering your own research questions. Remember that by using more than one method or data source you will strengthen your study's rigour and credibility ... this is known as triangulation.

References
- Cohen L, Manion L & Morrison K. (2000), Research Methods in Education. 5th edn. Routledge/Falmer, London.
- Gomm R & Davies C. (2000), Using Evidence in Health and Social Care, Sage, London.
- Robson C. (1993), Real World Research, Blackwell, Oxford.

Further information
Regarding relevant reading for quantitative methods, you might wish to look at:
- Bowling A. (2002) Research Methods in Health: investigating health and health services. (2nd. edn) Open University Press, Maidenhead.

And for qualitative approaches:
- Creswell JW. (2007) Qualitative Inquiry and Research Design. 2nd edn. Sage, London.

More generally, you might like to read:
- Blaxter L, Hughes C & Tight M. (1996), How to Research, Open University Press, Buckingham.
- Bowling A. (2002) Research Methods in Health: investigating health and health services. (2nd edn) Open University Press, Maidenhead.
- Creswell JW & Plano Clark V. (2007) Designing and Conducting Mixed Methods Research. Sage, California.
- Hicks CM. (1999) Research Methods for Clinical Therapists: Applied Project Design and Analysis. (3rd edn). Churchill and Livingstone – Harcourt Brace and Co. Edinburgh.
- O'Leary Z. (2004) The Essential Guide to Doing Research Sage, London. Wilkinson D. (ed.) (2000) The Researcher's Toolkit. Routledge/Falmer, London.

1.6 Research ethics and governance
Elizabeth White and Helen Hampson

The distinction between research ethics and research governance ~ frameworks ~ ethical review ~ NHS research ethics committees ~ research governance in social care ~ research, audit or service evaluation ~ implications of research governance procedures for therapists

This chapter outlines the Department of Health's *Research Governance Frameworks for Health and Social Care* (2005), covering all research activity in such settings. The process of obtaining ethical approval for research activity is described, and implications for therapists who are undertaking research are highlighted.

Research ethics and research governance: what's the difference?

Most therapists are aware of the need to obtain ethics approval for their research activity and may use the terms 'research ethics' and 'research governance' interchangeably. So what's the difference?

Research ethics refers to the principles that underpin ethical research. Two main perspectives inform ethical research: the need to provide the greatest benefit for the greatest number of people and the need to avoid doing harm to participants, researchers or others. These principles must inform your intended research activity, and your reasoning must also include consideration of the possible consequences of different courses of action.

Research governance can be defined as the broad range of regulations, principles and standards of good practice that exist to achieve and continuously improve research quality across all aspects of health and social care. These standards are in place to ensure that research activity meets the ethical principles described above. Your NHS Trust will have mechanisms in place to ensure that all research undertaken by its staff, with its patients, or on its premises, meets the standards required. Before considering any research you must contact your Trust's research and development (R&D) department to be sure that you are aware of all requirements and procedures.

Please be aware:
This book was written in 2008. Some of the details in this chapter may be out of date. Please seek advice from your Trust or your profession's Research and Development department.

Research governance frameworks

Your trust's research governance procedures will be designed to meet the *Research Governance Framework for Health and Social Care* (DoH 2005), which sets out the principles, requirements and standards that are expected of all people in health and social care settings who are undertaking, participating in or managing research in their organisation. This framework was developed to safeguard the public and to improve the quality of research by setting out the requirements for ethical approval and ensuring scientific rigour in all research activity. It is a statutory and legal requirement for health professionals to operate within the local approved governance systems.

Ethical review as part of research governance

In order to ensure that high standards are achieved in research activity, it is a requirement of the Department of Health that 'research involving patients, service users, care professionals or volunteers, or their organs, tissue or data, is reviewed independently to ensure it meets ethical standards' (DH 2005, p7). This process of review is undertaken by completing the application process of the relevant research ethics committee.

You will require approval from an NHS Research Ethics Committee for any research proposal that involves:
- patients and users of the NHS.
- research participants who are recruited because they are relatives or carers of NHS patients.
- patient data.
- NHS staff who are recruited as research participants by virtue of their professional role.

Ethical review of research is devolved within the UK, and policy responsibility for research ethics systems in the UK countries is:

England
Department of Health (Research and Development Directorate) **www.dh.gov.uk/en/Publicationsandstatistics/Publications/PublicationsPolicyAndGuidance/DH_4008777**

1.6

Northern Ireland
Department of Health, Social Services and Public Safety (Research and Development Office) **www.centralservicesagency.com/display/rdo_research_governance**

Scotland
Scottish Executive (Chief Scientist Office) **www.sehd.scot.nhs.uk/cso/Publications/ResGov/Framework/RGFEdTwo.pdf**

Wales
National Assembly for Wales (Welsh Office for Research and Development) **www.word.wales.gov.uk/content/governance/governance-e.htm**

NHS Research Ethics Committees (RECs)

Research ethics committees have been set up to scrutinise research proposals, to ensure that governance standards will be met by the proposed activity. Recent changes have taken place in the processes that govern ethical review of research proposals. The purpose of the changes is to increase the efficiency of the NHS systems, by seeking to ensure RECs only consider applications within their remit and that the level of review is appropriate to the ethical issues raised. You are advised to obtain information about current requirements from the National Research Ethics Service at **www.nres.npsa.nhs.uk**

In order to fulfil governance requirements, you will need to satisfy a number of conditions and you will find it very helpful to discuss what you will need to do with your supervisor or mentor. Trust R&D Officers and, in England, local Research and Development Support Units (RDSUs) are also a very good source of support.

An application for ethical approval should be made well in advance of your intended start date for the research. Before you apply, it is expected that you can provide written evidence that funding has been obtained for your project. Any research undertaken within the NHS must have a research sponsor, who assumes responsibility for ensuring an appropriate standard of research and that proper arrangements are in place for its conduct and reporting mechanisms. All proposals for health research must be subject to peer review and you can find further information about the peer review process on the NHS R&D Forum website at **www.rdforum.nhs.uk/workgroups/primary/pcinfoguide/4peerreview.htm**

All applications must be made on the NRES application form that is available at **www.nres.nprs.nhs.uk** Question-specific guidance is provided to assist you with completing your application, though you are recommended to seek advice from someone who has already successfully completed the application process. You will be expected to submit supporting documentation such as questionnaires or interview schedules with your application. Information sheets, consent forms and all recruitment materials will be reviewed by the committee.

NHS Research Ethics Committees usually meet on a monthly basis, and you are strongly advised to attend the meeting at which your proposal will be discussed. If you are present you will be able to answer any queries the committee may have, without further delaying the timescale for the response. A decision on your application will be made within 60 days from receipt of the application by the office, although you may be requested to make some amendments to your proposal.

For research in the NHS, you will also need to consider the requirement for local NHS R&D management approval for each site where the project will take place. Guidance on obtaining this approval is included with the NRES application form.

Research governance in social care

A different application process exists for research in social care. The Research Governance for Health and Social Care Framework resource pack, currently under review, aims to define good research practice in a local authority setting. Further information can be found at www.ssrg.org.uk/governance/index.asp. The document 'Guidelines for people who want approval for a multi-site social services project' can be obtained from **www.adass.org.uk/research/guidelines/guidelines.pdf**

Research, audit or service evaluation?

It can be difficult to identify whether the study you are proposing is research, audit or an evaluation of your service. All these activities may involve patients or their data, and may require the use of surveys or interviews. Ethical review is only mandatory for research, and it can be tempting to think of your proposed activity as audit or evaluation in order for it to seem more achievable. Being able to define the purpose of your work is essential.

1.6

Research is defined as *'the attempt to derive generalisable new knowledge by addressing clearly defined questions with systematic and rigorous methods.'* (DoH 2005). This definition emphasises that the research process aims to find out, by means of a systematic approach, what happens when a clinical approach or intervention is changed or explored. A quantitative or qualitative approach may be used to answer the research question, but the findings should be generalisable or at least transferable to a wider population than the sample or local service.

Clinical audit is a process that directly assesses services against a standard that has already been set, and provides a quality assurance mechanism for practice. Although patient contact may be involved in audit activity, and data collection methods such as surveys may be used, the process of audit does not produce generalisable knowledge, but aims to assess whether current practice meets required standards in the setting concerned.

Service evaluation is undertaken to identify information about a service, such as its cost and benefits, strengths and weaknesses. The process of evaluation may involve a range of data collection methods to record activities. It is often undertaken in response to identified local needs and is likely to involve a number of departments within an organisation.

The table opposite outlines key differences between research, audit and service evaluation.

Formal ethics approval is not required for activity that is clearly audit or service evaluation. However, if such activity raises significant ethical issues on which you would value REC advice you can contact the Chair of your local REC, enclosing a summary of your proposal.

Guidance to help you determine the category of your project can be obtained from the NHS R&D Forum at **http://www.rdforum.nhs.uk/docs/categorising_projects_guidance.doc**

	Research	Audit	Service evaluation
Purpose	Generate new knowledge	Assess if service meets given standard	Define current care
Methods	Quantitative – test a given hypothesis; Qualitative – explore theme using established methodology	Measure service against a stated standard	Measure service with no reference to a standard
	May involve a new treatment or allocation to a treatment group	Does not involve a new treatment or allocation to a treatment group	Does not involve a new treatment or allocation to a treatment group
Knowledge	Adds to the body of research knowledge	Provides knowledge about service being audited	Provides knowledge about service being evaluated
Ethics	Requires NRES approval	NRES review not generally required	NRES review not required
Dissemination	Publication output required	Usually reported locally	Local reporting

1.6

Implications of research governance procedures for therapists

Research governance procedures have been put in place to ensure that health and social care research meets the required ethical standards. Therapists now need to be aware that any research activity they undertake either in NHS or social care settings, with patients, carers, patient data or other health/social care professionals must have the required approvals in place before it can commence. This includes research you may undertake with your professional peers that is not within your workplace: for example, surveying members of a clinical interest group to determine the types of assessment they use.

It is important to identify in advance your research sponsor, and how your funding will be obtained. It is likely that your employing organisation will be the research sponsor for your work, and it is their responsibility to ensure that proper arrangements are in place for the management, monitoring and funding of the project. A clear dissemination plan is vital in order to share your findings widely, and this should preferably be via publication in a peer-reviewed journal. Note that most journals will require a statement of ethics approval to be included, and may refuse to publish your work if you cannot provide this evidence.

Be aware that you will need to obtain informed consent from your research participants, and that arrangements exist to protect vulnerable people or those who are unable to give consent. You will need to ensure the appropriate use, retention and protection of patient data.

Research governance procedures have had a significant impact on student research projects. Many pre-registration courses now do not offer students the opportunity to undertake their own research due to the time restrictions imposed by the need to gain ethical approval. Alternative strategies for involvement in research have resulted in the development of activities such as literature reviews, which denies students the opportunity for first-hand involvement in the research process. This may result in therapists who feel less confident in undertaking research once they have qualified.

Therapists need to be aware of the implications of undertaking research with professional colleagues. Workplace research may change the nature of the relationship you have with colleagues, as you may obtain information about people that would not normally be revealed. Think carefully about how you will handle this information and seek advice from your supervisor or mentor.

Don't let research ethics procedures put you off
The introduction of the research ethics review process has been seen as a barrier to undertaking clinical research, or research in health and social care settings. You will need to plan ahead in order to complete the requirements of the research governance frameworks, but achieving a successful application will give you confidence that your proposal demonstrates a good quality research project.

Reference
- Department of Health. (2005) Research Governance Framework for Health and Social Care, 2nd edn.
http://www.dh.gov.uk/PublicationsAndStatistics/Publications/PublicationsPolicyAndGuidance/PublicationsPolicyAndGuidanceArticle/fs/en?CONTENT_ID=4108962&chk=Wde1Tv

1.7 Collaboration and multidisciplinary research
Gail Mountain

Why research into multidisciplinary work? ~ who should do research into services ~ how does applied research differ? ~ which professions can be engaged in applied research? ~ involvement of end users and their carers ~ benefits of working with researchers from other backgrounds ~ learning from previous multidisciplinary research projects ~ getting involved

The whole is usually greater than the sum of the parts...

Background
There are many research questions which are specific to our professional practice; for example the effectiveness of physiotherapy interventions. Research neglect of allied health professions in the past resulted in very little evidence being generated to support practice. However, the situation is now improving to meet the demand for evidence-based practice and value for money.

Why research into multidisciplinary work?

Undertaking research to examine the individual contributions of certain professional groups is important but in the complex world of healthcare delivery, professionals rarely work in isolation. As a consequence, research questions are often concerned with services or issues that span a number of disciplines and are not the sole province of one profession.

Case example 1
Research regarding the effectiveness of rehabilitation for people following stroke will need to take the following into account:
- The service infrastructure.
- What is delivered to each patient and their carer and for how long.
- The contribution of each member of the multidisciplinary team.
- The overall service as experienced by the individual user and their carer.
- Measurement of the outcomes of rehabilitation for users and their carers.
- The costs of the service.

The impact of the whole multidisciplinary team and the environment within which they operate will have to be examined. In this example it would be difficult to separate the contributions of physiotherapists from that of other multidisciplinary team members.

Who should do research into services like rehabilitation?

From the late 1990s onwards, policy makers became increasingly aware of the potential value of rehabilitation services. This interest was accompanied by financial resources for research. One example of this was the research commissioned nationally into intermediate care services. The investment led to academic researchers becoming engaged in research into rehabilitation services. Projects similar to the one described in case example 1 have most frequently been undertaken by social scientists and other academic researchers. Thus, physiotherapists and others became the subjects of research rather than being engaged in the research process themselves. These projects often led to findings of a policy or academic orientation with less value for practice.

Most recently, the importance of applied research has been recognised. This examines questions of importance to those engaged in service delivery and to service users and their carers. This form of research often involves testing new interventions or ideas and is therefore ideally conducted by those with a good understanding of clinical practice and the needs of those using the service. As a consequence, the contribution which can be made by individuals with research training combined with a professional background such as physiotherapy, occupational therapy and nursing is being increasingly recognised.

How does applied research differ from other forms of research?

As applied research is about getting answers to questions rather than generating knowledge, it centralises the questions and concerns of those working in, and using services. These questions and concerns are then taken forward through the research process, which will utilise the clinical skills, experiences and professional networks of the researchers.

Case example 2
Research which aims to design functional and aesthetically attractive assistive technology for people with disabilities will need to take account of:
- The opinions of people with disabilities regarding what they need to help them as well as what they consider to be desirable.
- The views of their carers.
- The views of professionals who are responsible for prescribing assistive technologies.

1.7

These perspectives will be used to create prototype technologies by designers and technologists which users and carers and professionals will then be asked to test and give their feedback on. Designers will produce successive prototype devices until all stakeholders (users, carers and professionals) are in agreement about what is safe, fit for purpose and acceptable. This process is called an iterative design process.

Which professions can be engaged in applied research?

As case example 2 illustrates, conducting successful applied research will often involve a multidisciplinary team of researchers, from what can appear to be disparate professional groups. Researchers from professions like engineering, design and computing are realising that the involvement of clinical researchers can assist them to produce devices and other research products which people will want to use.

Case example 3
A large project to develop and test technology for home-based stroke rehabilitation was led by therapy researchers. It involved researchers from the following professions:
- Occupational therapy
- Physiotherapy
- Ergonomics
- Psychology
- Medical physics
- Movement science
- Informatics
- Engineering

The project also engaged with user advocacy groups and practitioners working in clinical practice and industry.

What about the involvement of end users and their carers?

One of the cornerstones of applied health research is the active involvement of people using health services and their carers. End users and their carers can be involved in research in the following ways:
- As commissioners of research; identifying research questions and advising on what should be funded.

- As advisors to research projects; for example as a member of a project steering group.
- As participants; providing information to researchers (this is the most familiar form of involvement).
- As researchers, following specific training; users can be involved in identifying research questions, collecting data and analysing data.

In case examples 2 and 3, users will be acting as participants and as advisors.

Case example 4
A project has been commissioned by the Expert Patient Programme (EPP) (the employees of which are all service users) to devise and test the feasibility of a self management programme for people with dementia and their carers. The project protocol is being written by an occupational therapist and a member of the EPP (who also has mental health problems). The feasibility of the programme of work will involve occupational therapy, psychology, psychiatry and user advocacy organisations. A person with dementia has agreed to join the steering group as an advisor.

More information about user involvement in research can be obtained from
www.involve.org.uk

What are the benefits of working with researchers from other backgrounds?

The benefits of well conducted, collaborative, multidisciplinary research are proven to be significant. It can enable a whole range of ideas and perspectives to be brought to bear to address a research problem. For example:
- The specific contributions of each discipline group.
- Sharing of methodological approaches.
- Expanding the communities to engage in the research.

Multidisciplinary research also challenges old ways of thinking. In particular, the involvement of end users in research can question both academic and professional perspectives.

1.7

What has been learnt from previous multidisciplinary research projects?

There a number of ways in which multidisciplinary research can be facilitated:
- Use of professional jargon must be limited. It is all too easy to lapse into professional jargon which is not understood by others outside the professional group. When a multidisciplinary group of researchers work together this effect can be magnified if a common language is not adopted.
- Good systems of communication must be established that are based in the use of a common language. The need to communicate and meet together on a regular basis increases with the greater diversity of groups included in any project.
- All researchers must maintain an open mind regarding what might be achieved.

These ways of working have much in common with good practice for involving users and carers.

How do I get involved?

The current focus upon applied multidisciplinary research and upon research which is focused upon helping people with long-term conditions to live independently means that it is has never been a better time for therapists to get involved. Involvement can include:
- Acting as a clinical partner; for example providing researchers with your clinical expertise, providing access to patients and assisting with the collection of data.
- Facilitating the dissemination and implementation of the results of research through professional networks.
- Assisting end users and carers to be involved in the research process.

Additionally, a small but increasing number of therapists will be motivated to become more centrally involved in the research process. This is a very rewarding and exciting area to work in. Some suggestions of how this might be achieved are as follows:
- Enrol for a higher degree in research so that you have the necessary academic credentials in addition to your clinical qualification.
- Attend multidisciplinary research conferences rather than professional events; one example is the Society for Research into Rehabilitation **(www.srr.org.uk)**.
- Keep appraised of current research in your area of interest and identify established

research groups.
- Engage in any opportunities to be a clinical partner in a research project, as previously described.
- Keep alert for small funding opportunities, particularly those from Research Councils.
- Allow yourself to think creatively of new ideas and possibilities for research.
- Identify researchers with the correct background to support you with funding applications and with other associated activities.
- Publish and get your name known.

Finally, remember...

Multidisciplinary groups of researchers who are engaged in applied research need people like you to make their ideas a working reality.

1.8 Applying for research funding
Sue Mawson

Funding schemes ~ targeting your research funding proposal ~ writing a proposal ~ factors for a successful submission ~ sources of further information

The aims of this chapter are to help you to:
- Describe various funding schemes for applied clinical research.
- Target your research proposals to the most appropriate scheme.
- Write your proposals for an appropriate submission.
- Explore factors that contribute to a successful submission.
- Provide sources of further information to help you develop high quality bids.

Sources of funding

In 2006 the Department of Health published the new NHS research strategy in a document entitled Best Research for Best Health. The strategy represented a huge change in the way research would be funded in England with the existing Research and Development levy (Support for Science and Priorities and Needs) ceasing from 2006/7. All current funding being withdrawn in a transition period to be completed in 2009/10. The National Institute of Health Research (NIHR) was created to hold all the research funding for programmes (Figure 1), infrastructure, faculty and systems.

Many of these grants, such as the programme grants and the Health Technology Assessment (HTA) and Service Delivery and Organisation (SDO) grants, are very prestigious awards for teams of researchers from the NHS and academia with impressive track records for research. They are not therefore appropriate for novice researchers. However, one NIHR programme is a responsive funding scheme called Research for Patient Benefit (RfPB). Allied health professionals are in a unique position to apply for this funding as they play a pivotal role providing front-line services and support to patients and carers. This enables them to have patient-focused insights into the kind of research described within the brief for the RfPB programme; research that will offer the greatest benefits to patient care.
www.nihr-ccf.org.uk/site/programmes/rfpb

The RfPB programme is:
- Located in the NIHR, coordinated through the central commissioning facility (CCF).
- Regionally implemented via ten regional commissioning panels covering government office regions.
- Budgeted proportionally to regional populations.

FIGURE 1

NIHR research
Translating research evidence into NHS practice

Proof of concept → Efficacy →

| Basic research (Biomedical, population, social sciences and engineering & technology) | Experimental medicine | Effectiveness and cost-effectiveness | Knowledge transfer for NHS | Adoption into the service |

- Research Centres
- Programme Grants
- Healthcare Technology Cooperatives
- Health Technology Assessment
- Service Delivery and Organisation
- **Research for Patient Benefit**
- Research for Innovation, Speculation and Creativity
- New & Emerging Applications of Technology
- Health Technology Devices
- NICE

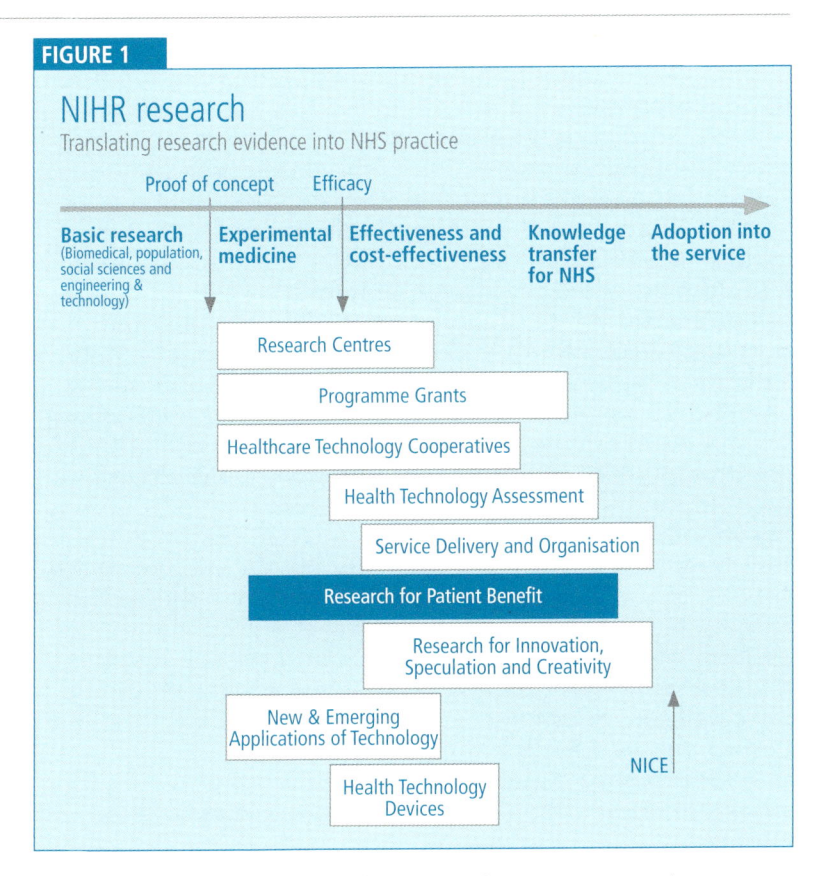

- Has a national budget that will build up to £25 million per annum over the next three years.
- Projects can last up to 36 months with a budget of up to £250,000.

The programme is intended to support research that is relevant to the day-to-day practice of health service staff and capable of showing a demonstrable impact on the health or healthcare of service users. Proposals that have emerged from interactions with patients/service user experience, and which have been developed with them and other agencies like voluntary bodies/public, are particularly welcomed. The funding is inclusive of qualitative and quantitative methods, unlike other funding streams such as the HTA programme, which is specifically for randomised controlled trials.

1.8

Research council grants
The Medical Research Council (MRC) is the most prestigious council designed to support biomedical science research in UK universities and NHS Trusts. Research grants do not cover research involving randomised trials of clinical treatments and the success rate is very low for the allied health professional (AHP) group. However, other research councils have proved very appropriate for a number of physiotherapy and occupational therapy researchers in the UK, for example, the Engineering and Physical Science Research Council (EPSRC). This body has a specific remit to support health research, particularly in the areas of quality of life for older people, technologies for rehabilitation of people with long-term conditions, dementia and nutrition. The EPSRC particularly favours multidisciplinary applications from engineers (medical physicists), computer scientists and healthcare professionals. While operating a responsive model funding stream, the council frequently has specific priority calls for health-related research. **www.epsrc.org** Depending on the type of research, other research councils may be relevant; links to all research council websites can be found at **http://www.rcuk.ac.uk/default.htm**

Charitable foundations
The BUPA Foundation is probably the most well known charitable organisation, funding research in the areas of surgery, preventative health, mental health in older people and health at work. Another source of funding is the Dunhill Medical Trust for research into elderly care, and the Health Foundation, which has various funding schemes. There are also disease-specific schemes such as the Multiple Sclerosis Society awards, which are very appropriate for AHP applications.

While there are a number of research funding sources, carefully targeting your application to the most appropriate scheme will inevitabley increase your chances of success.

Writing a successful proposal
While application forms may vary from funding stream to funding stream, there are some important points to consider when writing a proposal to undertake a research project. Most research and development departments in NHS organisations have guidelines for proposal writing, as all proposals have to undergo an 'independent scientific review' (ISR) prior to submission for ethics approval.

All proposals should have a literature review or background section, which provides the clinical and scientific justification for the study. Here you should include evidence of the clinical significance of the proposed work, whether this work has been carried out before, and how the proposal fits into the defined needs of the funding call. The application reviewer should feel confident that the research team are fully aware of relevant literature and ongoing studies in the area. When doing your literature review be mindful of the National Research Register that contains all current research activity **(http://www.nrr.nhs.uk/)**

There should then follow a clearly defined and answerable question based on the literature section. Your proposal should then contain a clear statement of objectives and a demonstration that the design of the project is appropriate to meet those objectives **(http://www.trentrdsu.org.uk).** For example if your objectives are to: *'Investigate patient views using a questionnaire'* or to *'Assess the effectiveness of a clinical specialists on patient care'*

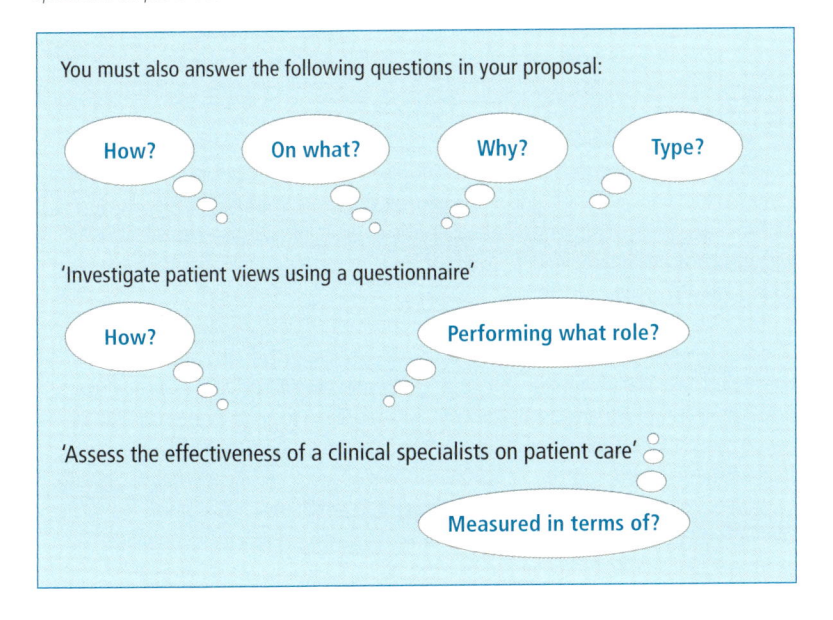

You must also answer the following questions in your proposal:

- How?
- On what?
- Why?
- Type?

'Investigate patient views using a questionnaire'

- How?
- Performing what role?

'Assess the effectiveness of a clinical specialists on patient care'

- Measured in terms of?

1.8

A successful bid will always provide a good justification for the research design chosen:

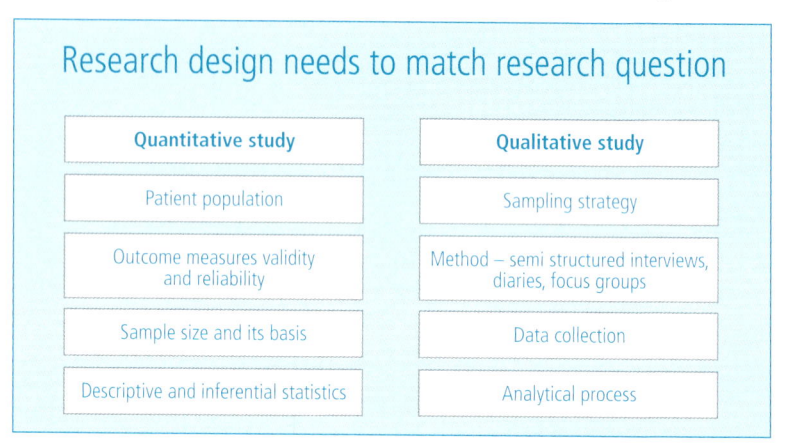

Research design needs to match research question

Quantitative study	Qualitative study
Patient population	Sampling strategy
Outcome measures validity and reliability	Method – semi structured interviews, diaries, focus groups
Sample size and its basis	Data collection
Descriptive and inferential statistics	Analytical process

You will also be expected to outline how the project will be managed. This should involve steering group meetings including not only the project team, but also someone to represent the patient group under investigation. For example, if you are studying the effects of a balance training intervention on falls frequency in a care home, it is quite useful to work with your local Age Concern group, inviting them to review your application and be on your project steering group.

One area where you will certainly need help is with costing the bid. NHS Trusts and universities have teams who can work on this with you and it is advisable to always seek help from the start. While you will know what you require in terms of a research assistant, travel costs and dissemination costs, the complexity lies in the need to identify 'excess treatment costs,' the annual 'up lift' for inflation and of course the thorny issue of overheads. Most NHS organisations will have their own overhead, which usually runs at around 30 per cent; however, universities now have to use what is called a full economic cost model (FEC), which virtually doubles the staffing costs in the bid.

In your application you should also demonstrate that current research governance frameworks and procedures for ethics approval have been followed. For more information on these processes, see the following websites:
- National Research Ethics Service based within the National Patient Safety Agency **(http://www.nres.npsa.nhs.uk)**
- Department of Health for Research Governance Framework **(http://www.dh.gov.**

uk/Policyandguidance/researchanddevelopment/research
- Medical Research Council Guidance on ethics and best practice **(http://www.mrc.ac.uk/index/publications/publications-ethics**)

Ten top tips for successful bid writing

1 Read the application form and guidance notes many times, highlighting with a marker pen key words and the submission deadline.
2 Don't reinvent the wheel: the reviewers are all experts in the field and they will be up to date with current and previous work in the area.
3 Seriously consider public/patient involvement **(http://www.invo.org.uk)**.
4 Work with academic partners: most reviewers will expect this. However don't just go for the 'big names'; you must clearly identify the role of the partners in the project.
5 Get advice from a statistician and a health economist if appropriate, and tell the reviewer in the text where and how the advice was sought.
6 When describing the dissemination process, don't just talk about conferences and journal articles. Try to demonstrate how you will influence not only practitioners, but also policy makers.
7 Make sure your costings are correct.
8 Don't dismiss pilot work, pre-pilot work or clinical audits that may have been done prior to your application. Tell the reader what you have done in the background section.
9 Outcomes should be patient focused where possible, using well-designed outcome measures.
10 Don't panic! There are plenty of people to help, many of whom need your clinical expertise to provide important clinical questions.

Sources of further information
- http://www.nihr.ac.uk
- http://www.mrc.ac.uk
- http://www.rdinfo.org.uk

Each strategic health authority has within it a research support unit (soon to become 'project support units') and these can be hugely helpful in writing research applications: see **http://www.trentrdsu.org.uk** for an example of an RSU. Also remember that your local university may have a clinical trial support unit (CTSU) and that local healthcare organisations may be able to offer help and support in writing a good, scientifically rigorous and potential clinically beneficial research application.

1.9 Collecting good quality data (quantative, qualitative and mixed)
Anne Bruton and Caroline Ellis-Hill

GIGO ~ data collection ~ sampling procedures ~ information to be collected ~ recording the data ~ data storage

GIGO

The term garbage in, garbage out (GIGO) is one of the great truisms of the computer age, meaning that if unreliable, inaccurate or inappropriate data are entered into any system, the resulting output will inevitably be unreliable, inaccurate or inappropriate. In other words, the quality of your analysis, findings and ultimate conclusions will be directly dependent on the quality of the data you collect.

Data collection

Collecting data is sometimes considered the most enjoyable or exciting stage of research and can involve anything from observing behaviour to conducting interviews, sending out questionnaires or taking measurements. There are a few general points:
- It is better to collect small amounts of good quality data than large amounts of rubbish.
- Seek advice – consider having an advisory group for the project.
- Set up and keep to a timetable for the study.
- Maintain good, clear records and organise your data (that is coded, dated and so on).
- Be clear as to why you are collecting data and how you are going to use the data you collect. Check back to your research questions to be sure that analysing the data you collect will produce some answers to your questions.
- Beware of any biases: yours and/or other researchers'.
- Be aware that you can affect something just by observing/measuring it – hence the need for rigorous standardisation. Your data collection procedure must follow the protocol approved by the ethics committee.
- Set up clear procedures for managing the data (for example entering databases, filing paper records).
- Be scrupulous in your approach to the data, even if it is not coming up with the answers you wanted or expected.
- Minimise the number of people who have access to your data.

Sampling procedures

In quantitative research, the aim is to sample individuals who will be representative of a particular population so that results can be generalisable. The population to be studied is therefore carefully defined and described and, ideally, a random sample is attempted that is each individual in the population has an equal chance of being selected. Sample size is determined using statistical formulae to ensure inferences can be drawn with some confidence. In qualitative research the aim is to generate data from a specific group of participants and describe the context (for example setting, participant characteristics, interviewer) in sufficient detail to allow others to judge the theoretical generalisability of the data. The qualitative researcher often selects a small number of individuals to provide in-depth information. The exact number will depend on the approach used for example narrative, case study, grounded theory, ethnography, phenomenology.

Information to be collected

Whether you choose quantitative, qualitative or mixed methods of data collection will depend on the research question and the focus of the research, that is a researcher's or participant's perspective. If you want to know how much flexion a new knee replacement gives women aged 65–70 years, then you need to collect numerical measurements for example of joint angles. If you want to know about their experience of having a knee replacement, then you need some form of discourse. Mixed method studies use both qualitative and quantitative techniques, either as distinct components or explicitly integrated. Quantitative techniques obtain numerical data to measure performance or attitude, which can be subjected to statistical tests. Qualitative techniques, on the other hand, obtain data about experiences and feelings. Do not assume that quantitative data are more reliable or valid than qualitative data, this is not the case – it all depends on how they are collected, recorded and interpreted.

Recording the data

Data collection involves systematically gathering and recording this information so that it can be stored and analysed by an individual or by a team. In quantitative research, ideally a different person should analyse the data from the one who collected it, to avoid bias and potential for inappropriate data manipulation. If this is not possible, data should be coded so that the person measuring it is blinded to its source. In qualitative research it is

1.9

helpful if the same person does both. Always pilot your research protocol to see if it as practicable as you think it is, and to identify any areas that need change.

- Quantitative data
- Qualitative data
- Mixed methods data

Quantitative data
- A standardised, detailed step-by-step data collection procedure from recruitment to completion should be written and adhered to consistently.
- Any equipment/measurement tool/questionnaire used should be both reliable and valid. It should have previously been validated for the specific population you wish to study. If your work is exploratory/ground-breaking this may not be possible, but you should then be doing reliability/validity studies before using the tool in your research. Precision is not the same as accuracy – just because you can measure something to three decimal places does not make it 'true' (or useful).
- Any equipment/measurement tool used should be calibrated and serviced regularly so that performance is optimal and the results can be trusted.
- A standard operating procedure (a specific guide for usage) should be produced for all equipment (in some cases this might be the manufacturer's instruction manual).
- All raw data should be recorded and retained in indexed laboratory notebooks with permanent binding and numbered pages or in an electronic notebook dedicated to that purpose. Records in notebooks should be entered as soon as possible after the data are collected, identified and dated. Subsequent modifications or additions to records should also be clearly identified and dated.

Qualitative data
- Ensure that your data collection and analysis are consistent with your underlying methodological and philosophical assumptions.
- A detailed step-by-step data collection procedure from recruitment to completion should be written and adhered to consistently.
- As well as transcriptions from either interviews or observations, fieldnotes are helpful in describing the context of the interaction. A reflective diary can be used to note your personal influence on data collection and analysis.
- Make sure that any recording equipment is functioning correctly. Check regularly.
- Individuals vary in their ability to articulate their thoughts and ideas. Practise and

refine your interview techniques, to facilitate participants' accounts and to create quality data with them.
- Aim to begin analysing your data as soon as possible after collection.
- Increase credibility by asking more than one person to analyse a small amount of data to ensure that alternative interpretations are not overlooked and can be included in the analysis.

Mixed methods data

In a mixed method study, quantitative and qualitative data will either be collected concurrently or sequentially. Concurrent strategies have been employed to validate one form of data with another, to transform data for comparison, or to address different types of questions. Sequential strategies involve collecting data in an iterative process whereby data collected in one phase contribute to data collected in the next. Qualitative data will provide a deeper understanding of survey responses, and statistical analysis can be used to provide detailed assessment of patterns of responses. However, the analytic process of combining qualitative and survey data can be time consuming and expensive.
- Whether you use concurrent or sequential methods, you need to use rigorous quantitative and qualitative procedures, as above.
- It is common practice (but not essential) to use the same group of participants for both the quantitative and qualitative components, to make convergence/comparison of the data more straightforward; however, sample sizes are likely to differ.
- If data are collected concurrently, be aware of potential for bias whereby one form of data collection may confound data from another form.
- If data are collected sequentially, you have to decide how you will select results from one phase for examination in more detail in another phase, for example what criteria will you use for this choice?

Data storage

Maintaining confidentiality of all data collected during any research project is essential. All personal information should be encoded or anonymised as far as is possible and be consistent with the needs of the study. If you are not going to use the information, do not collect and record it.

Appropriate and secure storage of all primary data is of paramount importance, for the protection of your participants and you as a researcher. Clear rights and levels of access to the data should be specified at the outset of any research project. Data should

1.9

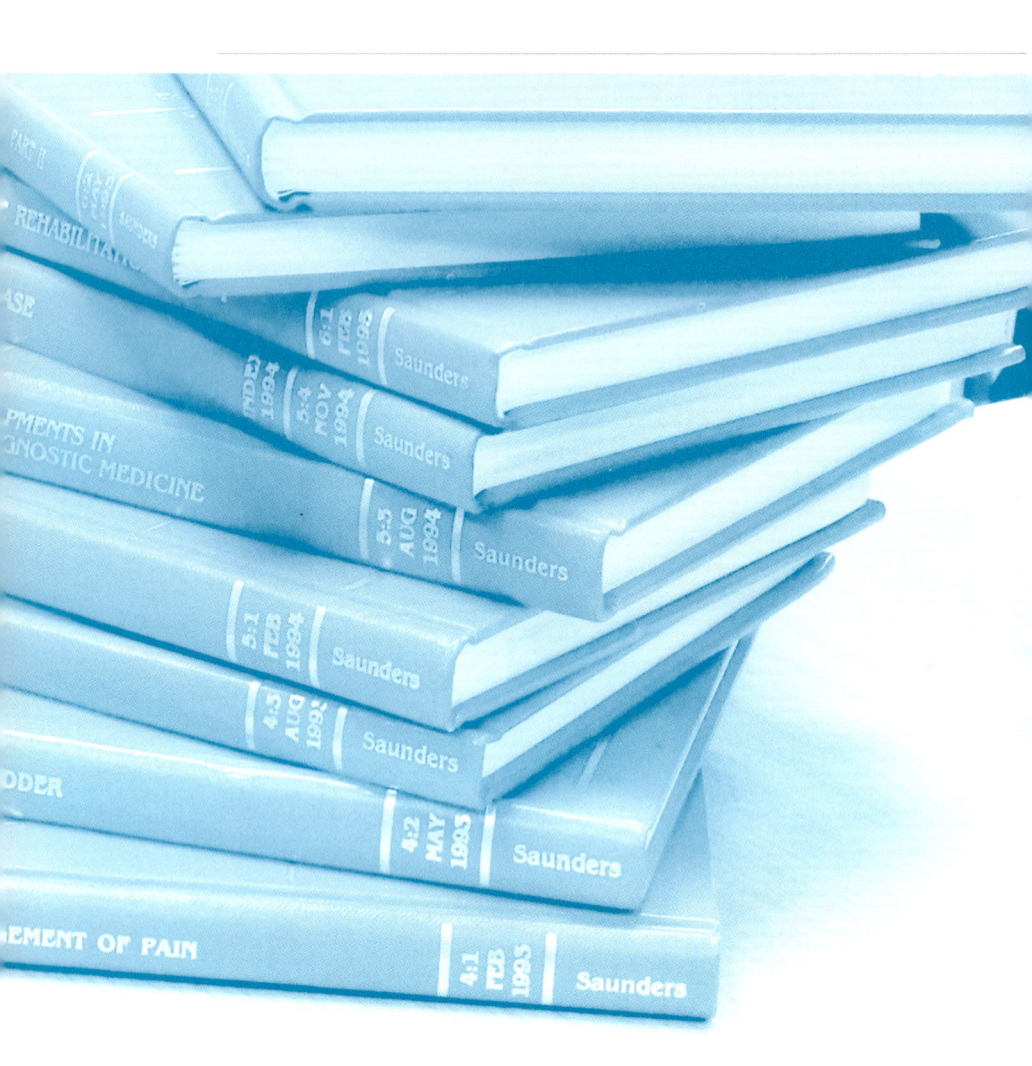

be stored safely with appropriate back up and contingency plans in the event of loss, damage or unauthorised access to the data. Wherever possible a complete duplicate set of the original data should be retained. Your data must be retained and archived in their original raw form, as a precaution, particularly as published results may be challenged by others. Your institution will have guidelines stating for how long this should be (often 10–15 years).

And finally...

Some key questions to ask yourself while collecting data:
- Why am I collecting these data?
- Am I sure that I am recording reliable and valid information?
- Am I following the standardised protocol approved by an ethics committee?
- Are my data being securely stored during the data collection process?

Further information
- Creswell JW. (2002) Research Design: Qualitative, Quantitative, and Mixed Methods Approaches (2nd Edn). Sage Publications, Inc, Thousand Oaks, CA.
- Sim J and Wright C. (2000) Research in Health Care: Concepts, Designs and Methods. Nelson Thornes Ltd, Cheltenham.
- Jenkins S et al (1997) The Researching Therapist: A Practical Guide to Planning, Performing and Communicating Research. Churchill Livingstone, New York.
- Sapsford R and Judd V. (2006) Data Collection and Analysis (2nd Edition). Sage Publications Ltd, London.

1.10 Analysis of data
Julius Sim

Data preparation ~ choosing a strategy for quantitative analysis ~ reporting quantitative analyses ~ choosing a strategy for qualitative analysis ~ conclusion

Introduction

The process of data analysis should tie in logically with the philosophical perspective within which a study is situated, the research questions or hypotheses that have been developed, the overall design of the study, and the specific methods of data collection that are to be employed. It is important, therefore, to take account of the intended method of analysis when first planning a study, so that data are collected in a sufficient form, and maybe also in sufficient quantity, to facilitate subsequent analysis, and in particular to ensure that certain methods of analysis are not foreclosed by inappropriate decisions at the level of study design or data collection.

Data preparation

Appropriate data preparation is a prerequisite for any type of analysis. Quantitative data should be entered into an appropriate statistical package. This should preferably be a specialist statistical package (for example MINITAB, SPSS, STATA) rather than a more general spreadsheet package with statistical functions (for example Excel), as the analytical capabilities of the latter may be limited. The data must be cleaned (for example incorrect or out-of-range values corrected, missing values identified) and, where appropriate, recoded and transformed (for example items in a multi-item scale added to provide a summative score).

Whereas there is little merit in conducting quantitative analyses by hand, a reasoned choice may be made between manual and computer-aided analysis for qualitative data analysis, according to the particular approach to be taken to the analysis, the quantity of data to be analysed, and the personal preference of the researcher. In either case, most qualitative data will require transcription. N-Vivo is a popular package for qualitative analysis, but others are available. Whichever is chosen, it is important to remember that the interpretive element of analysis must remain with the researcher, and that while the computer can facilitate, and to some extent enhance, this process, it cannot replace it.

Choosing a strategy for quantitative analysis

For quantitative data, appropriate descriptive analyses will always be required; when hypotheses are to be tested or when sample data ('statistics') are used to estimate corresponding properties of the population ('parameters'), inferential analyses will be required in addition.

In either case, clarity as to the level of measurement – viz. nominal, ordinal, interval, or ratio – of each variable is required. The distinction between interval and ratio measurement is rarely of concern in terms of selecting techniques and procedures, but other distinctions – such as between nominal and ordinal, or between ordinal and interval/ratio – are normally important.

Some important principles relating to descriptive analysis are:
- Descriptive summaries and graphics must be chosen with regard to the level of measurement of the data (Table 1).
- As a measure of central tendency, the mean and median should be accompanied by a measure of dispersion (standard deviation and interquartile range, respectively).
- Percentages should be accompanied by the numbers on which they are based.
- Be wary of presenting percentages of percentages, as readers will find these confusing.
- Use graphs judiciously, and only where these will be more informative than a textual presentation.
- Use terminology carefully – for example specify a 'mode', 'mean' or 'median', not an 'average', as these are all types of average; distinguish between the situation in which there are two or more variables and that in which there are two or more sets of scores on a single variable.

For inferential analysis, it is important to determine the statistical hypotheses to be tested before inspecting the data. This will help to limit the number of analyses and prevent 'data dredging'. This, in turn, will control the Type 1 error rate (the 'false positive' rate, or more technically, the probability that one or more null hypotheses will be incorrectly rejected).

1.10

TABLE 1

Examples of appropriate descriptive statistics and graphs for differing levels of measurement

Level of measurement	Appropriate descriptive statistics	Appropriate graphical display
Nominal	Mode	Bar chart; pie chart
Ordinal	Median; interquartile range	Bar chart; boxplot
Interval/ratio	Mean; standard deviation (median and interquartile range for skewed distibutions)	Histogram; stem-and-leaf plot; error plot; boxplot; bar chart (for counts or percentages, but never for mean values)

Other important decisions to be made in advance include:
- The probability value that marks the threshold for statistical significance, for example $p \leq 0.05$. This is referred to as alpha, and represents the probability of a Type 1 error.
- Whether sets of values are related or unrelated. If two or more sets of scores come from the same sample of individuals, or from groups that have been matched on one or more characteristics, values are related; if they come from two or more unmatched groups of individuals, they are unrelated.
- Whether a parametric or (when available) a nonparametric test is to be used (Table 2). Parametric tests make certain assumptions as to the nature and distribution of the data to which they are applied; nonparametric tests make fewer or no such assumptions. These assumptions should be checked before a choice is made between these types of test.
- Whether a 1-sided (1-tailed) or a 2-sided (2-tailed) hypothesis test is to be used. A 2-tailed test seeks a significant effect in whatever direction, whereas a 1-tailed test focuses on an effect in a specified direction. 1-tailed tests are problematic on a number of grounds, and are best avoided.

The power of a statistical test is the probability that it will detect as significant an effect that exists in the sample (more technically, the probability of rejecting the null hypothesis when it is false). Sample size is the principal determinant of statistical power, and should be determined at the outset of a study and built into its design. At the point of analysis, therefore, sample size is usually pre-determined. Be wary, however, of planning analyses (for example on subgroups) that are likely to have little power, as these will probably be

TABLE 2
Examples of some parametric tests and their nonparametric counterparts

Parametric test	Nonparametric test
Pearson correlation coefficient	Spearman correlation coefficient
Unrelated t test	Wilcoxon rank sum test
Related t test	Wilcoxon signed-ranks test
Oneway analysis of variance	Kruskal Wallis test
Repeated measures analysis of variance	Friedman test
Factorial analysis of variance	None

inconclusive. The failure to reject a false null hypothesis is referred to as a Type 2 error, and is the complement of statistical power, for example if a study has power of 0.90, there is a Type 2 error rate of 0.10.

When designing a quantitative study that is likely to involve more than the most basic analyses, it is worth seeking the advice of a statistician. This should be done at an early stage, as decisions made in relation to the design of a study will have implications for its analysis, and inappropriate choices at this point may either facilitate or foreclose subsequent analyses.

Reporting quantitative analyses

When reporting the results of hypothesis tests, certain principles should be followed:
- State the value of alpha to be used at the outset (for example 'statistical significance was set at $p \leq 0.05$, 2-tailed'), and then report actual p values from individual tests.
- When reporting statistical tests, you should report the test statistic, the degrees of freedom or sample size (as appropriate), and the p value – for example for a t test: 't = 2.347; df = 742; p = 0.019', or for a correlation coefficient: 'r = 0.097, n = 239, p = 0.136'.
- As well as the information from a statistical test, give the magnitude and direction of an effect, for example '... the mean score in Group A exceeded that in Group B (mean difference = 7.9)...'.

- Use accurate terminology – for example a hypothesis is either 'rejected' or 'retained', but it is not 'proved'; procedures, not data, should be described as parametric or nonparametric; be clear as to whether findings are statistically significant, clinically significant, both, or neither.

Where summaries such as means or proportions are presented as estimates of the corresponding parameter in the population, a confidence interval (CI) should be quoted. This indicates a range of plausible values for the population value, given that this is unlikely to correspond precisely to the sample estimate. However, CIs are not appropriate for a simple descriptive summary of the sample.

Note that individual journals may have specific requirements as to how statistical analyses are reported. For statistical tests, for example, a journal may not require the test statistic to be reported, only the p value.

Choosing a strategy for qualitative analysis

Different approaches exist to the analysis of qualitative data and it is neither desirable nor possible to specify a single appropriate method. As a general principle, the method of analysis selected should relate to the philosophical and theoretical perspectives and the methodological principles that underlie the study.

That said, it is possible to distinguish two common, broad approaches to qualitative data analysis:

Thematic content analysis: this involves a search for recurrent ideas or meanings in the data, which are then placed within themes or categories. The purpose is to identify elements of commonality within the data that can be used to construct an interpretive framework. A balance is struck between establishing such commonality and maintaining a sense of the individuality of particular participants' accounts.

Narrative analysis: the emphasis here is more on constructing a 'story' within the accounts of individual participants. Often, the aim is to explore a person's biography, or life history, through one or more extended one-to-one interviews. While theoretical connections are often made between narratives, the concern is less with identifying commonality than in thematic content analysis.

Although, as previously mentioned, there is no orthodoxy in the analysis of qualitative data, the following principles command a reasonable degree of acceptance:
- Avoid a simple statement of the data, and attempt to move to a more interpretive (though not unduly speculative) level of analysis, so as to generate insights with implications for a theoretical understanding of the issues or topics being researched.
- Provide sufficient raw data, for example in the form of quotations, to justify the interpretation of the data. It may be useful to link quotations to (anonymised) individuals.
- Be alert to, and report, data that may not fit emerging insights; it is easy otherwise only to find what you expect to see in terms of conclusions that have already been formulated.
- Place the data analysis within a broader social, institutional or environmental context, so that the analysis does not become 'disembodied' from its natural context. In the process of contextualising your data, be careful to preserve the anonymity of individual participants.
- Strive for reflexivity – an acknowledgment of the role played by the researcher, with his or her particular experiences, perceptions and values, in both the creation and analysis of qualitative data.
- If appropriate, refine or 'test' your interpretation of the data with one or more other researchers. Similarly, your insights can be shared with your informants, to see if they find them to be a plausible interpretation of what they said ('respondent validation').

Conclusion

Good data analysis relies on a judicious and theoretically informed choice of appropriate methods. Above all, it must link to the questions or hypotheses that form the basis of the study, and the results of data analysis must be presented in a way that is clear and intelligible.

Further information
- Argyrous G. (2005) Statistics for Research, with a Guide to SPSS, 2nd edn. Sage, London.
- Armitage P, Berry G, Matthews JNS. (2002) Statistical Methods in Medical Research, 4th edn. Blackwell Science, Oxford.
- Banister P, Burman E, Parker I, Taylor M, Tindall C. (1994) Qualitative Methods in Psychology: a Research Guide. Open University Press, Buckingham, 142–159.
- Freeman JV, Walters SJ, Campbell MJ. (2007) How to Display Data. Blackwell, Oxford.
- Roberts B. (2002) Biographical Research. Open University Press, Buckingham.
- Silverman D. (2004) Doing Qualitative Research: a Practical Handbook, 2nd edn. Sage, London.
- Sim J, Wright C. (2000) Research in Health Care: Concepts, Designs and Methods. Nelson Thornes, Cheltenham.
- Strauss A, Corbin J. (2008) Basics of Qualitative Research: Techniques and Procedures for Developing Grounded Theory. 3rd edn. Sage, Thousand Oaks.

1.11 Strategies for dissemination of research
Krysia Dziedzic

The research question ~ the protocol ~ research findings ~ research publication ~ dissemination to the wider audience ~ implementation ~ knowledge translation

The aim of this chapter is to present a range of strategies that could be used to disseminate research. The strategies are based on different stages of the research process with examples to illustrate each stage.

Introduction

Dissemination is an important element of the research process and should not be reserved only for the conference style dissemination of results. Dissemination is about effective communication of research findings to a range of key stakeholders, for example fellow colleagues, health professionals, researchers, patients, the public, policymakers and commissioners.

Figure 1 illustrates the different stages of a research cycle and it is within each of the stages that the dissemination of research should be considered. The cycle is particularly relevant to the randomised controlled trial but qualitative designs, and other quantitative designs such as epidemiological studies and observational studies, could be mapped on a similar cycle. Each stage of the research process will be illustrated by examples of dissemination activity.

The research question

Once a research question has been formulated then dissemination of the question to key stakeholders is essential. John Tukey said that 'an approximate answer to the right question is worth a great deal more than an exact answer to the wrong question'. To ensure that the right question is being addressed, it is important to share this question with service managers and the research team, including statisticians and health economists, health professionals and user representatives, that is patients and the public.

The key elements to discuss are the population to be recruited to the study, the intervention to be delivered, the comparator against which the intervention will be tested and the outcome measures.

FIGURE 1

Stages of the research cycle

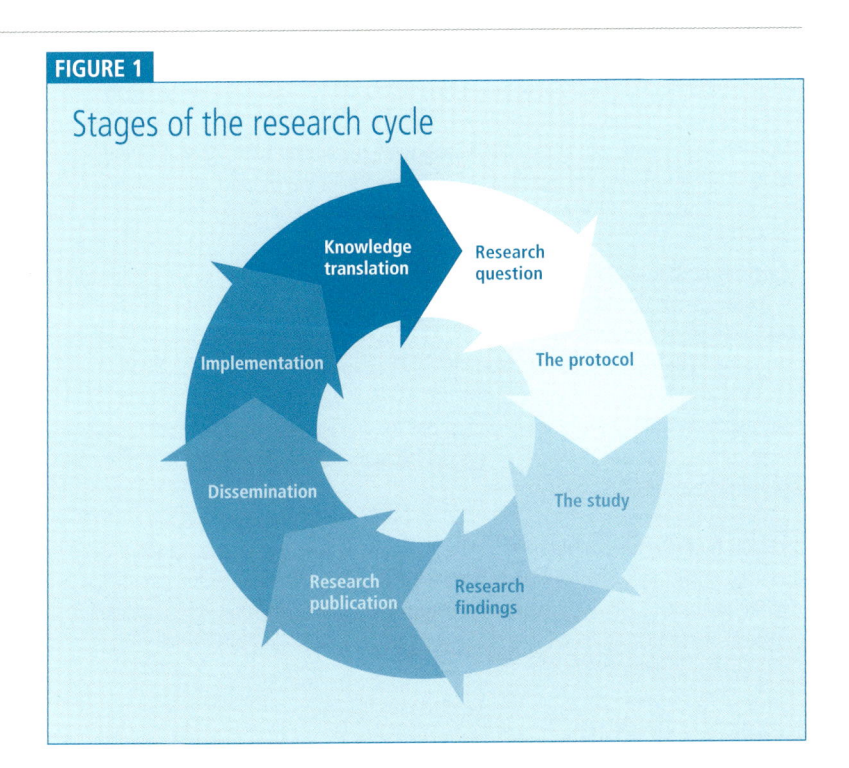

- Knowledge translation
- Research question
- The protocol
- The study
- Research findings
- Research publication
- Dissemination
- Implementation

One way of disseminating the research question is by developing a clinical advisory group that comprises patients, members of the public, health professionals and researchers. A small workshop or oral presentation with discussion of the issues may be the best way to gain consensus on the importance of the question and to determine whether this is the right question to be addressed at this time.

The protocol

The protocol will describe how the research question will be answered. The protocol can be disseminated via posters to clinical departments and general practices. It has become more common to publish the study protocol, for example, in open access journals (Peat et al, 2006; Lamb et al, 2007; Myers et al, 2007).

1.11

The study

Throughout the study, particularly if it is long-term, it is important to disseminate the progress of the study to key individuals. Dissemination of the conduct of the study will ensure best practice in undertaking the research.

A brief newsletter can be an effective way to communicate with practitioners, to provide an update on such matters as the number of participants recruited to the study, and any additional information of importance. This will help to keep the momentum of the study going and, in particular, assist recruitment, which is always the biggest challenge.

Clinical advisory group meetings or workshops for practitioners can be held throughout the study to update people about progress, highlight areas of good practice and discuss issues that may be causing difficulties.

A clinical trial may have a Data Monitoring Committee, who will require six-monthly updates on the trial's progress. This will take the form of a trial monitoring report. The Arthritis Research Campaign **(www.arc.org.uk)** has a template that is recommended for use in arc-funded studies.

Research findings

Analysis of the study will produce the research findings. These will be discussed initially within the research team, for example by the principal investigator, study co-ordinator, statistician and health economist. Once the research team is clear that all the appropriate analyses have been undertaken then the research findings need to be disseminated to the wider group, which may include other members of the research team, health professionals involved, therapy managers and participant representatives. Dissemination to this group will enhance the interpretation of the research findings prior to further dissemination.

A common method used to disseminate findings is presentation at local, national or international conferences. Follow the conference instructions carefully to increase the chances of having an abstract accepted. The choice is often oral or poster presentation and clear guidance on the format for these will be given. An example of an abstract template and a poster template can be seen in Figures 2 and 3. It is not usual to submit the same abstract to multiple conferences. However, should you wish to submit the same research

FIGURE 2

Example template of an abstract

Title: The XXXX Study

Authors: 1,
1. Affiliations

Background

Methods

Results

Conclusions

Funding and acknowledgements

to more than one conference, contact the organising committee or refer to their guidance on what they will and will not accept. Different aspects of the same research study can be presented in different abstracts. The challenge is to identify which conference to target with which piece of work. Feedback at the conference will enable further discussion about the interpretation of the findings and help to prepare the study for publication.

FIGURE 3

Institutions logos   Title
Funding logos   Authors[1]
                       1. Affiliations

  Introduction
                  Methods: Trial follow-up
                                              Table/graph of results
  Objectives
                       Flow chart
                                              Conclusion
  Methods
                                              Acknowledgements
                                              • The participants
                                              • The physiotherapists
                                              • The GPs and their staff
                                              • Funding agency
Methods: Trial recruitment
             Contact details email and address

1.11

A medical illustration department should be consulted early on for help with the production of posters. Images and other material will need to be prepared in a format that will enable reproduction. Handouts relating to a poster can be distributed at the conference, but it is usual to decline any requests by the conference organisers for presentations to be put on a website or CD for universal distribution; such requests should be declined if this is unpublished work.

Always practise your oral presentations with friends and colleagues before the conference. Get them to pose you questions that might be asked. Novice presenters may wish to consider targeting specific conferences that have a reputation for being very supportive and encouraging for 'first timers', for example, the Physiotherapy Research Society.

Remember that attendance at conferences costs money and opportunities to fund this should be sought through various channels.

Research publication

A guide for publication is covered in the following chapter. In choosing the right journal to submit to, consider seeking advice to make the right choice and plan carefully for submission.

There is a whole range of journals that might be considered when deciding where to publish. High quality international peer reviewed journals have high impact factors (high quality and citation) but also have very high rejection rates. The manuscripts accepted here often have multiple authors. Authors may have contributed to the conception and design of the study, the writing of the original research proposal, the data collection, the analysis and interpretation of data, the drafting of the manuscript, the process of revising it critically and its final approval. A national journal may be more applicable if your findings are not relevant to an international audience. A journal targeting specific healthcare practitioners may be preferred if you want to convey your findings to groups of health professionals in particular.

Good physiotherapy evidence depends on the quality of the research and communicating the findings to others. However the skill of writing papers is frequently overlooked. Many published studies are reported poorly despite the efforts of researchers, editors and peer reviewers. Reporting guidelines exist (for example CONSORT, STARD) but they are still not widely used by physiotherapists. A new international initiative, the EQUATOR

Network, aims to improve the reliability of publications by enhancing the reporting of health research **(http://www.equator-network.org/).**

Once your study has been published in a scientific journal then the next step of dissemination can be undertaken.

Dissemination to the wider audience

If the study has had external funding, the funding body may wish to disseminate the findings to a lay audience and may contact you for a press release. This press release will be sent to professional newsletters and local press to generate interest about the study. Writing a lay perspective of the research findings will be useful. The dissemination of results to the research participants can be undertaken through a variety of means, for example, posters in general practices and letters to individual participants.

Implementation

At this stage your research publication may be picked up by authors of clinical evidence papers, clinical practice guidelines, evidence-based practice groups (for example Stevenson et al, 2007) and opinion leaders. Practitioners and researchers often work closely to appraise the evidence and generate local practice guidelines. No single method works best, but active methods are far more effective than passive ones.

Knowledge translation

There has been a recent move to consider how knowledge can be translated from evidence into practice and to shorten the journey between the dissemination of research findings and changes in practice (Davis et al, 2003).

One of the key differences in dissemination at this level is dialogue with policy makers and commissioners. These stakeholders are used to action and require simple, straightforward messages that can be interpreted speedily into a plan for service delivery.

Knowledge translation is an interdisciplinary process. It will engage researchers from a variety of backgrounds, as knowledge translation requires methodologically diverse designs. It involves the public, patients, clinicians and researchers. The Canadian government has been very keen to address this, and models of good practice are being adopted in the UK.

Conclusion

Dissemination strategies need to be considered at all stages of the research process in order to ensure effective translation of research into clinical practice. Different strategies include posters, oral presentations, workshops, focus groups, publications in scientific journals, publications in the popular press and communication with a wide range of stakeholders in the health economy, including commissioners of research, clinical opinion leaders, patients and the public. Optimal dissemination requires a team approach and a multiplicity of strategies.

The stages of the research cycle can be useful to signpost the important elements of dissemination. Different research designs may need a different approach and this should also be considered.

The novice researcher may begin in an arena of relative security and then with experience progress to presenting at international conferences and publishing in a range of journals to reach different audiences.

Acknowledgements

Thanks to Hilary Jones for assistance with the manuscript for this chapter.

Reference list
- Davis D, Evans M, Jadad A, Perrier L, Rath D, Ryan D, Sibbald G, Straus S, Rappolt S, Wowk M, Zwarenstein M (2003). The case for knowledge translation: shortening the journey from evidence to effect. British Medical Journal 327(7405): 33-5.

- Lamb SE, Lall R, Hansen Z, Withers EJ, Griffiths FE, Szczepura A, Barlow J, Underwood MR (2007). The back skills training trial (BeST) team; design considerations in a clinical trial of a cognitive behavioural intervention for the management of low back pain in primary care: back skills training trial. BMC Musculoskeletal Disorders 8: 14.

- Myers H, Nicholls E, Handy J, Peat G, Thomas E, Duncan R, Wood L, Marshall M, Tyson C, Hay E, Dziedzic K (2007). The clinical assessment study of the hand (CAS-HA): a prospective study of musculoskeletal hand problems in the general population. BMC Musculoskeletal Disorders 8: 85.

- Peat G, Thomas E, Handy J, Wood L, Dziedzic K, Myers H, Wilkie R, Duncan R, Hay E, Hill J, Lacey R, Croft P (2006). The knee clinical assessment study-CAS(K). A prospective study of knee pain and knee osteoarthritis in the general population: baseline recruitment and retention at 18 months. BMC Musculoskeletal Disorders 7: 30.

- Stevenson K, Bird L, Sarigiovannis P, Dziedzic K, Foster NE, Graham C (2007). A new multidisciplinary approach to integrating best evidence into musculoskeletal practice. Journal of Evaluation in Clinical Practice 13(5): 703-8.

Further information:
http://www.nice.org.uk/usingguidance/implementationtools/howtoguide/barrierstochange.jsp

1.12 Writing for publication
Philippa Lyon

Types of article ~ selecting a journal ~ writing and editing ~ submission and the peer review process

Types of article

- The case study
- Publication from a research thesis
- The research paper
- The review or systematic review

Case study
A case study is a detailed description of the application of a treatment to a specific clinical use. This type of article enables you to write directly about your practice, and can be particularly useful as a first step if you are relatively new to writing for publication.

Publishing from a thesis
If you have completed a masters' or doctoral thesis, there may be the potential to produce articles from it. Thesis material for an article needs to be carefully selected and prepared so that it stands as a piece of work in its own right, not just as an 'excerpt' from your thesis.

Research paper
Original research into a particular topic or question should be presented as a scientific research paper. This requires a range of basic research skills. A research paper should always include an introduction, a description of the methods you have used, the results and a discussion of the significance of the results.

Systematic review
A review examines the evidence on a particular topic or question by first identifying what evidence exists, then summarising and providing a critique of it. Systematic reviews are considered to be the best quality, and are based on a specific methodology and structure. Reviews do not simply provide descriptions of existing material, but offer analysis, including issues and implications for practice and further research.

Selecting a journal

- Fitting the journal scope and style
- Assessing journal quality
- Advice and guidance

Scope
Each journal has a specific scope, for example a particular clinical specialty or methodology, and a description of this is normally included in the journal. Some journals also favour particular types of articles. It is very important to take account of this to ensure you are producing your article for the most appropriate publication. Journals also employ a range of different house styles and layouts and you need to prepare your article with this in mind. Scanning through sample article titles and abstracts in a particular journal, and consulting the journal's instructions to authors, will help you identify whether your article is likely to 'fit'.

Quality
Journal quality is variable. The most widely used quantitative measure of journal quality is the 'impact factor'. This measures the citations to science and social science journals as indexed and calculated by the Institute of Scientific Information (ISI). Impact factors are published annually and whilst there is some debate about their reliability, they are extensively used as indicators of the quality of a journal and the research contained within it.

Advice and support
When considering which journal to submit an article to, in addition to seeking advice from experienced researchers or clinical/special interest groups, you can also try sending an abstract to the editor for feedback on its suitability.

1.12

Writing and editing

- Planning
- Writing techniques
- Writing style
- Editing

Planning

Clarify the precise aim of your article before you begin to write. If you are fairly new to writing for publication, try to find a clinical or educational mentor to provide you with some support and advice.

Check the style of the journal you have selected and the format required for your article type. You need to be clear before you start on:
- word limits (for each section and for the whole article).
- title and keywords guidance.
- abstract style.
- format, including headings/sub-headings for the article.
- referencing style.

If you are writing as part of a team, be clear what each member of the team is responsible for in the writing up, what the deadlines are and how co-authors will be listed in the final article. The order of co-author names is sometimes organised according to the degree of involvement by each author and journals can ask for a covering letter giving details of this, or for a contributors' statement, as part of the article.

Before writing, estimate roughly how many words you can apportion to each section of your article. Ensure also that you have sufficient knowledge of literature on the topic in question, and that you can make reference to this where relevant.

Writing techniques

If you have not had extensive experience of writing for publication, read through a selection of articles in your chosen journal and consider the style of writing used. This can vary in the degree of formality and amount of background knowledge assumed.

Using the guidance provided by the journal on article format, make a plan of the key points to be made in your piece against the required headings and sub-headings.

Consider who the readers of your chosen journal are, and keep their needs in mind as you write. Ensure all sections of your article follow on logically from one another. Read through drafts of your work as you write and redraft to improve the overall coherence.

Writing style
Keep sentences as short and clear as possible.

In many cases, journals will expect articles to be written from an impersonal standpoint, using the third person and the past tense (for example 'The research project showed that ..' rather than 'I showed that ..'). However, you should always check the specific requirements in the instructions to authors, as there are some variations, especially in relation to the preferred style for writing up qualitative as opposed to quantitative research.

Avoid jargon, and be consistent in the use of abbreviations and referencing (journal house style).

Editing
The author is responsible for checking the spelling, grammar and accuracy of an article submitted to a journal. In particular, the editing process should pick up:
- any inaccurate statements or assumptions.
- points that have been inadequately explained or justified.
- sections or points that are in an illogical order.
- typographical or spelling mistakes.
- grammatical errors.
- redundant words and phrases.
- any sources or funding bodies that have not been acknowledged.
- any copyright permissions that have not been fully cleared.
- any missing, incomplete or inconsistent references.
- any of the journal's style or format requirements that have not been met.

Submission and peer review

Submission to journals is usually electronic, via a customised submission system, but you should always check the requirements of the particular journal you are submitting to. Check that you provide everything required and ensure everything is in the required format and clearly labelled.

1.12

The process of peer review (see Figure 1)
Following an acknowledgment from the journal you have submitted your article to, the journal editor will send your manuscript to reviewers. There will usually be at least two reviewers.

Once the reviewers have considered your manuscript, they will make a report and one of three recommendations to the journal editor. Note that:
- It is possible for an article to be rejected outright if it is of insufficient quality, is not offering anything new, has a poor standard of presentation or does not sit within the journal's scope. In this case, it is possible to take account of the criticisms and consider revising and resubmitting your article to an alternative journal.
- Many articles are accepted subject to major or minor amendments.
- Articles are very rarely accepted unconditionally.

If you have been asked to make amendments to your article, these should be completed and returned to the editor with a summary of the changes made in a covering letter. If any of the requested changes have not been made, the reasons for this should also be explained. Very complex or poorly executed changes may be passed by the editor back to the reviewers for a final decision.

Once a final decision has been made to publish an article, a letter of acceptance is sent by the editor. At this point, the author is usually asked to sign over copyright to the journal and to check the proofs.

A final note
It is worth remembering that the whole process, from submission through to publication, can be very lengthy. It is also important to note that if you are rejected, while it can be very disappointing, the process of writing and submitting for publication is valuable for your continuing professional development, and the reports provided by peer reviewers on your work can give you extremely useful information for your future growth as a researcher.

Further information
- Many academic journal publishing companies have guides to writing for publication – check websites for the publisher of your target journal.
- There are searchable databases of journals on the ISI Web of Knowledge Service for UK Education. This may be accessible via an educational institution or your employer, and can be found at: **http://wok.mimas.ac.uk/**.

FIGURE 1

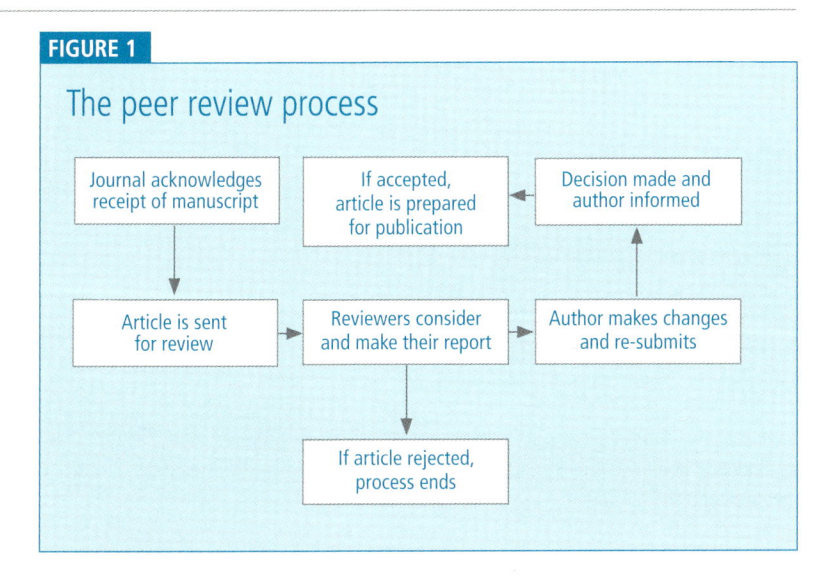

The peer review process

```
Journal acknowledges       If accepted,              Decision made and
receipt of manuscript  →   article is prepared   ←   author informed
                           for publication
        ↓                                                   ↑
Article is sent       →    Reviewers consider     →    Author makes changes
for review                 and make their report        and re-submits
                                    ↓
                           If article rejected,
                           process ends
```

- There are further useful guides to writing up and writing for publication in the following texts:
- Denscombe M. 2003 'Writing up the research', Chapter 15, p284-298, The Good Research Guide, 2nd edition Open University Press, Maidenhead.
- Hicks, C M. 1999 'Writing up the research for publication', p115-122, Research Methods for Clinical Therapists, 3rd edition Churchill Livingstone, Edinburgh.

1.13 Writing for scientific publications: tips from an editor
Michele Harms

Format ~ language ~ illustrations ~ revisions ~ data reduction ~ permissions ~ authorship ~ peer review

Presentation

- Format and structure
- Title
- Language, grammar and translation
- Figures and illustrations

Having a paper published in a scientific, and preferably peer-reviewed journal is the aspiration of most researchers and scientists. Publications add to the credibility of both the work and the authors.

Format and structure
When submitting a paper for publication, first impressions are very important and a paper can stand or fall by its abstract. Take as much care over the front page of your manuscript as you would over your CV. Some editors make their initial decision to reject based on the abstract alone, consequently if the author has failed to follow the guidelines to authors about the length, structure or content, the paper can be rejected without further consideration. If the guidelines for authors ask for a structured abstract under the headings 'Objectives, Design, Participants and so on' it would be inadvisable to submit an abstract with the headings 'Background, Introduction, Results, Conclusion'.

An article that is visually pleasing, has a sound and logical structure and contains the appropriate information under well thought-out headings will help convince the editor and reviewers that you, the author, are both conscientious and professional. Authors can fall foul of journal preferences, sometimes in spite of conducting a sound study. While many reviewers and editors may look at the value of the work beyond these issues and allow resubmission of a revised paper, you should not depend upon this and endeavour to submit your best work from the outset.

Title
Before submission, consider the title of the paper very carefully. The PICO (population/intervention/comparison/outcome) format can help ensure that all the important pieces

of information are contained (see Table 1). This acronym helps you to combine the key aspects of a clinical scenario into a title, a clinical question or a research topic for formulating a proposal, which can also be used to define a search strategy.

TABLE 1

Patient/Population	Intervention	Comparison/ Control	Outcome
Parkinson's disease	Balance training	Exercise	Frequency of falls
Chronic low back pain	Cognitive behavioural therapy	No treatment	Quality of life

Your title might be: Is cognitive behavioural therapy more effective than no treatment in improving quality of life in people with a history of chronic low back pain? This format will only apply to certain styles of paper and it is worth scanning the titles of your intended journal to ensure your title conforms to an appropriate style. It is also a useful technique to clarify the style of paper at the end of the title, for example: Physical therapy to reduce the effect of respiratory viruses: a systematic review.

Language, grammar and translation

Many journals support the campaign for plain English (**www.plainenglish.co.uk**), and encourage contributors to use straightforward, uncomplicated language. Authors can make the mistake of describing what can be complex approaches or methodologies, in equally complex language. If they haven't given up already, the reader may struggle to understand the language without even contemplating the underlying concept that the author wishes to convey. If English is not your first language, consider a co-author whose first language is English, or at least ask someone to proofread your paper, who not only has the language skills but understands the subject matter. Try to make your article concise and make every word count. Think hard about what really needs to be in the paper to get your message across accurately and what can be left out. Balance the word count so that the paper is not 'discussion heavy' or focused solely on the introduction. Give serious consideration to collaboration with a senior author, so you can benefit from their expertise in writing for publication. The ability to write clearly and concisely can take many years to perfect.

1.13

Illustrations and figures

Graphs tend to be submitted in a standard format. Generally they are produced in a software package like Excel (Microsoft Corporation, Redmond, USA) or SPSS (SPSS Inc Chicago USA). While the format can be tailored appropriately to the data, papers are often submitted with graphs in the default format which may be due to the author's unfamiliarity with the software. This is most easily seen in graphs where, for example, the accuracy of measurement is to the nearest whole number, yet the axis of the graph is labelled to two decimal places, the default format for some software. Familiarity with the software will allow modifications to be made reasonably easily. To see how the graph will look in published form, it should be reduced to the size it will appear in print. You will then be able to judge whether the axis labels and titles are in an appropriate sized font to be legible when reduced to the final size.

The quality of illustrations is also important. A photograph by a colleague without attention to lighting, focus, framing and background for instance, gives an unprofessional feel which tends to reflect upon the paper as a whole. The advent of digital cameras and electronic manipulation has resulted in an improvement in image quality. However it may still be advisable to use an experienced photographer. Alternatively, if a high quality image cannot be obtained, consider asking an illustrator to provide a suitable diagram or possibly omit the image altogether.

Considerations in the writing process

- Read, re-draft and revise
- Data reduction
- Permissions
- Authorship
- Peer review as a positive experience

Read, re-draft and revise

One of the most frustrating lessons to learn from writing a paper is the endless cycle of re-writing, revising and editing when preparing a manuscript for submission. Once the author has 'finished' this cycle it is wise to ask several people to read the paper and comment honestly. It takes a good friend or colleague to critique frankly and their criticisms should be met with gratitude rather than annoyance! Ask a colleague from a different background to read your paper and comment on areas they don't understand. While someone outside the target audience may not understand subject specific information, they should be able to comment on ease of reading, explanation of key concepts and so on. Ask a peer, someone from the target audience, to read your manuscript to determine suitability and level of understanding. Ask an experienced author to comment and make recommendations. Try to be as technically correct as possible – not only by conforming to the guidelines for authors, but by painstakingly checking reference lists are complete and accurate.

Data reduction
Where data are part of a paper, the key to presentation is simplicity and transparency. Complex data analyses are occasionally justified, but they are often hard to understand and can mask true patterns (or lack of) in the data. Present summarised data in the simplest form to introduce the results – before and after scores are often more telling than change scores for example. Means or medians with appropriate measures of confidence are universally acceptable. If the data is not normally distributed, or is ordinal (ordered categories) then use nonparametric analyses. When there is justification for more complex tests, these should not preclude the presentation of the basic, transparent data.

Permissions
Before submitting a paper, you will need to consider whether any approvals are necessary. Where photographs of individuals are to be included, you may need to obtain their written consent. Covering the eyes is not sufficient to assure anonymity. Case histories generally require the written permission of the person featured, stating that they have seen the paper and agree that it can be submitted for publication, even in the absence of a photograph. This is because they often deal with rare or unusual cases, again making it difficult to guarantee anonymity. Where illustrations are reproduced from other sources, permission from the copyright holder should be sought.

The point at which a paper is submitted for publication is not the appropriate time to seek ethical approval for a study. On occasions where papers are submitted and the appropriate approval for the research has not been granted, it may be possible for the author to obtain retrospective approval. However, any research involving human subjects requires approval or waiver from an appropriate ethical body and this should be granted before undertaking the work and not at the point of submission for publication.

1.13

Authorship
Most journals have fairly strict guidelines to define who qualifies as an author. This is based on making a significant contribution to the paper and on standing as guarantor for the integrity of the work. If you are new to writing for publication, consider working with a senior author. Not only will you benefit from their experience, but their involvement will add credibility to your work.

Seeing peer review as a positive experience
Receiving reviews can be a disheartening experience, as even the most seasoned author will tell you. But it is important to remember that it is rare to receive such useful feedback as that provided through peer review. If you receive full reviews, try not to take the criticism personally but appreciate that the reviewers have not only read, but taken time to understand and comment upon your work.

When receiving criticism of a paper you have nurtured, the first response is often to be defensive. When the reviewer misunderstands a point, it is natural to blame them for their ignorance, rather than to accept that you have written something that is not easily understood. A second reading will often show you what you left out, or why it has been misinterpreted.

There are courses on writing for publication which take the new author through this iterative process. Guidelines are also available for authors and mentors to guide a programme of academic writing in order to produce a succinct paper (Murray 2007). However, writing is a skill that can be learnt and developed and with time, having nurtured your ability to write convincing and cohesive arguments, you will also have the skills to become a reviewer.

Reference
- Murray R, Newton M. 2007 Facilitating writing for publication, Physiotherapy, doi:10.1016/j.physio.2007.06.004.

Further information
- Lyon, P. (2007) Hints and tips on how to write for publication in academic and professional journals Elsevier: Oxford.
  http://www.writingforpublication.com/

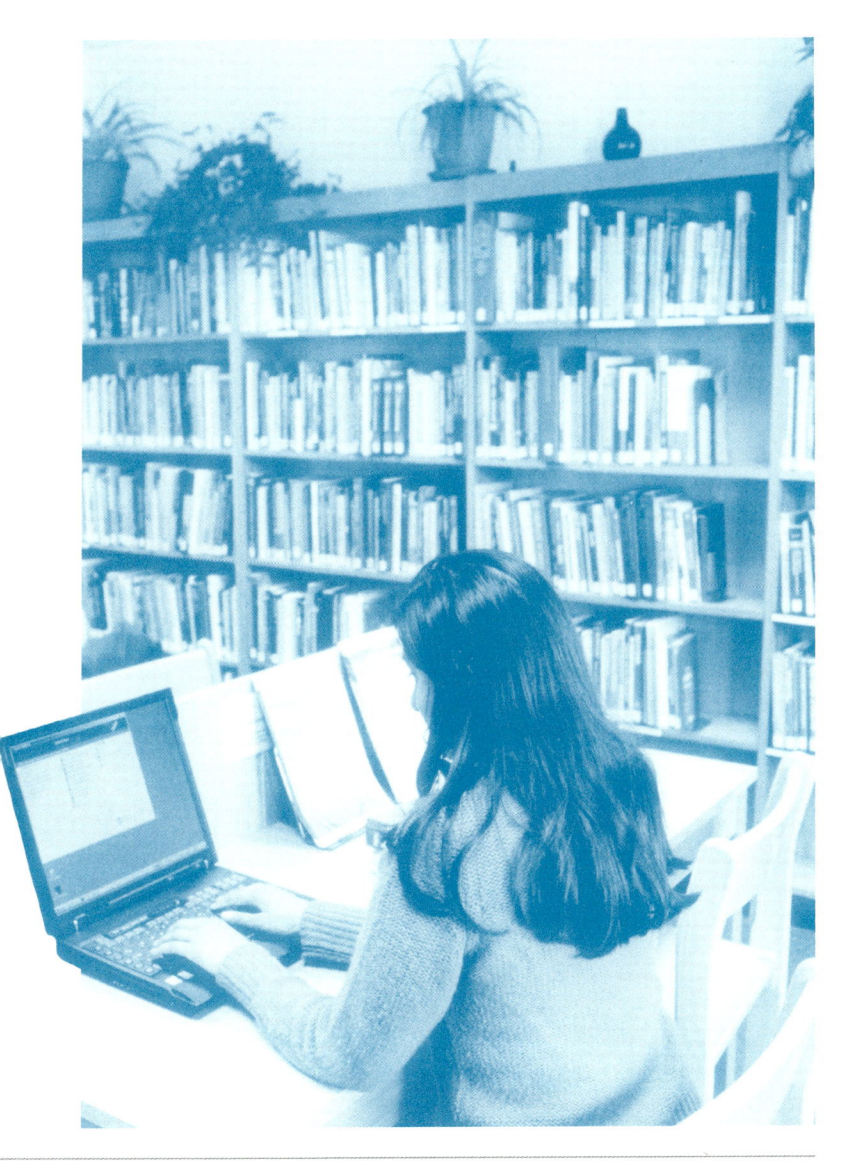

1.14 Integrating your own research into practice
Mindy Cairns

Implementation versus dissemination ~ change management ~ barriers to evidence-based practice ~ re-evaluation ~ evaluation of implementation ~ further information

This chapter covers the issues surrounding integrating your own, and other people's, research into routine clinical practice. It builds on previous chapters detailing the concepts of dissemination and evidence-based practice and provides guidance for how research can be successfully integrated into practice including change management and implementation, associated barriers and re-evaluation.

So you are finally there, the ultimate goal; project finished, you have your answers; now what? Far from being the end of the journey in terms of research this is where the hard work begins. Whether returning to clinical practice after completing your BSc, MSc or PhD research project or after completion of a work-based project, the issue is always the same; how do you integrate research into practice?

Implementation versus dissemination

At the end of your research process there is always the inevitable 'dissemination strategy' (see chapter 1.11). However dissemination implies a somewhat passive process where research findings simply reach practitioners as opposed to implementation where findings are actually incorporated into practice. Put simply dissemination is about raising the awareness of research findings while implementation is concerned with change in practice (NHS, 1999; Herbert et al, 2001). Interventions designed to change the behaviours of healthcare workers to be more in line with the current evidence base can be categorised into two broad headings:

- **Educational approaches**
  Educational approaches can be passive, such as distribution of educational material, conferences, didactic lectures or manual and electronic reminders, or more active such as educational outreach work, interactive education and audit and feedback.

- **Organisational or financially based approaches**
  Including financial incentives or penalties, to promote adherence to guidelines/evidence based treatment processes (Freemantle, 2000).

Educational interventions generally have shown little effect on change in behaviour with multifaceted approaches incorporating a number of modalities recommended to

be more effective than single modalities (Grimshaw et al, 2004). When attempting to translate research into practice, consensus from researchers has suggested 10 potentially effective elements to successful implementation (van Tulder et al, 2002):
1   Clear and strong evidence base.
2   Content of the messages.
3   Clear messages.
4   Consistent messages across professions.
5   Communication with stakeholders.
6   Clear sense of ownership (multiprofessional and public included).
7   Charismatic leadership.
8   Continuity of care as a background issue.
9   Continuous education: specific and practical.
10 Continuous evaluation.

These elements may be useful to consider when integrating your own research into practice but fundamentally what is central to successful integration is that the desired change in behaviour is successfully achieved.

Summary

- Passive dissemination alone is unlikely to result in changed behaviour.
- No one intervention/implementation strategy is effective under all conditions.
- Multifaceted interventions which target barriers to change are most likely to be effective.

(NHS, 1999)

Change management

As identified above, the aim of dissemination and implementation is to change behaviours; put simply you may want therapists to stop what they are doing and modify their practice according to your research findings. In attempting to translate your work into clinical practice you are requiring colleagues to undertake a process of change, and to sign up to your research. Numerous theories of change management exist and although a full commentary on all models is outside the scope of this chapter,

1.14

summary knowledge of key concepts will be of use when attempting to integrate your research into practice.

Introduction

- Translating theory into practice relies on a process of change.
- Change can often be unwelcome, challenging and disturbing for many.
- Understanding the concepts of change management may help integrating research into practice.

Three types of change processes have been identified that are helpful as an overview to change management (Ackerman, 1997; Iles & Sutherland, 2001):

- **Developmental change**
  - Aims to enhance or correct aspects of an organisation (or practice) often by building on existing strengths.
  - Can be either planned or 'emerge' and is incremental.

- **Planned or transitional change**
  - Aims to achieve a known state that is different from the present one and is planned but episodic.

- **Transformational change**
  - Major changes in the assumption of organisation and individuals; may result in significant changes in structure, processes, culture and strategy within the organisation.
  - A process of continuing learning and encouraging new patterns of thinking.

(Miller, 2000)

A frequently cited model of transitional change is that suggested by Lewin (1951) and incorporates three distinct phases: un-freezing, moving and re-freezing. Initially an individual or organization, for instance an outpatient department, identifies or realises that there is a need for change. This may be in response to the publication of compelling new research evidence (hopefully your own!), triggered by patient or carer feedback or by questions raised within daily clinical practice. This stage is unfreezing. The second stage, moving, requires active involvement of the individuals or group to change behaviour for example clinical practice, in order to successfully achieve the agreed goal. The final stage, re-freezing is achieved when the desired change in practice has occurred and a new culture has been established (Lewin, 1951).

Anecdotally, many therapists returning to clinical practice after completing further studies or research report difficulties in engaging colleagues to adopt changes in practice in response to research findings. In this case a developmental change process could be an ideal starting point when attempting to translate your own research findings into practice. As research knowledge is certainly a 'strength' within the workplace, a developmental change process may allow therapists to initiate and develop a more evidence-based culture within the workplace. Similarly the continual learning and encouraging new patterns of thinking embedded within transformational change would seem to fit very closely with continuing professional development and the development of clinical reasoning that is key to professional autonomy.

Summary

- The specific processes by which change occurs will vary in different situations.
- Change incorporates a number of reasoned steps and normally one step needs to be fully achieved before the next one can be successful.
- Identifying potential barriers to change is essential for successful, sustained change.

So if the theory of dissemination, implementation and change management in relation to research findings is relatively clear, why is research evidence not always used in practice?

Barriers – why is evidence not used in practice?

It is widely accepted that there are distinct gaps between what research findings indicate is 'best practice' and actual clinical practice. Certainly in the area of low back pain, numerous published evidence-based guidelines (CSAG, 1994; RCGP, 1996;

1.14

Burton & Waddell, 1998; Koes et al, 2001; Staal et al, 2003; van Tulder et al, 2004) have not resulted in the translation of research into actual clinical practice (Foster et al, 1999; Gracey et al, 2002; Rebain et al, 2003). The causes for these gaps have been reasonably well researched and a number of 'barriers' to the implementation of research findings identified:

Barriers to evidence-based practice

Research skills
- limited critical appraisal skills.
- limited understanding of statistics.
- limited understanding of the research process.

Implementation of research findings
- poor dissemination/accessibility of research findings.
- lack of clarity of the anticipated outcomes of using research.

Organisational culture
- lack of time and/or culture of doing rather than questioning.
- lack of resources.
- lack of access to training.
- resistance to change.
- perceived lack of support from other health professionals and/or managers.

Individuals and organisations will respond differently to proposed changes and will also identify different barriers. Assessment tools such as the BARRIERS to Research Utilization Scale (Funk et al, 1995) are available to assist in identifying potential barriers. As implementation strategies designed to address specific barriers are more likely to be effective than a generic approach (NHS, 1999), identifying potential barriers should be top of the list when implementing research!

Re-evaluation

So, you have identified and addressed the barriers to change, actively implemented your research findings, it is now important to evaluate (NHS, 1999; Herbert et al, 2001). How you do this will depend on the anticipated effect of any change (see Figure 1).

It may be that your aim was to increase the use of evidence in practice (process). Alternatively, or hopefully in addition, your aim may be improved patient outcome (outcome). It is important to be clear regarding your aims as integrating research into practice may have differential effects on process and outcome. For example, active strategies to implement clinical guidelines on physiotherapy for low back pain have demonstrated moderate effects on adherence to the guidelines (Bekkering et al, 2005a) but showed no effect on patient outcome (Bekkering et al, 2005b).

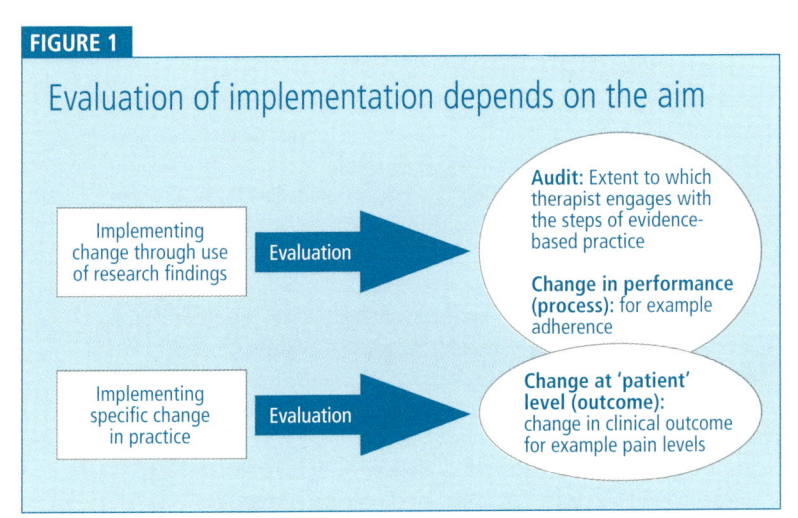

FIGURE 1
Evaluation of implementation depends on the aim

Implementing change through use of research findings → Evaluation →
- **Audit:** Extent to which therapist engages with the steps of evidence-based practice
- **Change in performance (process):** for example adherence

Implementing specific change in practice → Evaluation →
- **Change at 'patient' level (outcome):** change in clinical outcome for example pain levels

Change can often be challenging and changing practice is no exception. In the era of evidence-based practice it is important that therapists embrace new research and incorporate it into their own practice. An understanding of the stages of change management should help facilitate the integration of research into practice. Acknowledging and identifying potential obstacles or barriers to change is vital if change is to be successfully achieved. Just as Rome wasn't built in a day, so change isn't made in a day. The integration of research into practice should be viewed as a process and as such will take time, but should be worth it in the end.

Reference list
- Ackerman L. (1997) Development, transition or transformation: the question of change in organisations. Jossey Bass, San Francisco.
- Bekkering GE, Hendriks HJ, van Tulder MW, Knol DL, Hoeijenbos M, Oostendorp RA

1.14

& Bouter LM. (2005a) Effect on the process of care of an active strategy to implement clinical guidelines on physiotherapy for low back pain: a cluster randomised controlled trial. Quality and Safety in Healthcare. 14, 107-112.
- Bekkering GE, van Tulder MW, Hendriks EJ, Koopmanschap MA, Knol DL, Bouter LM & Oostendorp RA. (2005b) Implementation of clinical guidelines on physical therapy for patients with low back pain: randomized trial comparing patient outcomes after a standard and active implementation strategy. Physical Therapy. 85, 544-555.
- Burton A & Waddell G. (1998) Clinical guidelines in the management of low back pain. Baillieres Clinical Rheumatology. 12, 17-35.
- CSAG. (1994) Clinical Standards Advisory Group on Low Back Pain. Her Majesty's Stationary Office. London.
- Foster NE, Thompson KA, Baxter GD & Allen JM. (1999) Management of nonspecific low back pain by physiotherapists in Britain and Ireland. A descriptive questionnaire of current clinical practice. Spine 24, 1332-1342.
- Freemantle N. (2000) Implementation strategies. Family Practitioner 17 Suppl 1, S7-10.
- Funk SG, Tornquist EM & Champagne MT. (1995) Barriers and facilitators of research utilization. An integrative review. Nursing Clinics of North America 30, 395-407.
- Gracey JH, McDonough SM & Baxter GD. (2002) Physiotherapy management of low back pain: a survey of current practice in northern Ireland. Spine 27, 406-411.
- Grimshaw JM, Thomas RE, MacLennan G, Fraser C, Ramsay CR, Vale L, Whitty P, Eccles MP, Matowe L, Shirran L, Wensing M, Dijkstra R & Donaldson C. (2004) Effectiveness and efficiency of guideline dissemination and implementation strategies. Health Technology Assessment 8, iii-iv, 1-72.
- Herbert R, Sherrington C, Maher C & Moseley A. (2001) Evidence-based practice - imperfect but necessary. Physiotherapy Theory and Practice 17.
- Iles V & Sutherland K. (2001) Managing Change in the NHS: A review for healthcare managers, professionals and researchers: National Co-ordinating Centre for NHS Service Delivery and Organisation R&D.
- Koes BW, van Tulder MW, Ostelo R, Kim Burton A & Waddell G. (2001) Clinical guidelines for the management of low back pain in primary care: an international comparison. Spine 26, 2504-2513; discussion 2513-2504.
- Lewin K. (1951) Field Theory in Social Science. Harper Row. New York.
- Miller D. (2000) Leading an empowered organisation. Creative Healthcare Management Inc. Minneapolis, USA.
- NHS. (1999) NHS Centre for Reviews and Dissemination: Getting evidence into practice Effective Health Care 5.
- RCGP. (1996) Clinical guidelines for the management of acute low back pain. Royal College of General Practitioners. London.

- Rebain R, Baxter G & McDonough S. (2003) The passive straight leg raising test in the diagnosis and treatment of lumbar disc herniation: a survey of United Kingdom osteopathic opinion and clinical practice. Spine 28, 1717-1724.
- Staal JB, Hlobil H, van Tulder MW, Waddell G, Burton AK, Koes BW & van Mechelen W. (2003) Occupational health guidelines for the management of low back pain: an international comparison. Occupational and Environment Medicine. 60, 618-626.
- van Tulder MW, Croft PR, van Splunteren P, Miedema HS, Underwood MR, Hendriks HJ, Wyatt ME & Borkan JM. (2002) Disseminating and implementing the results of back pain research in primary care. Spine 27, E121-127.
- van Tulder MW, Tuut M, Pennick V, Bombardier C & Assendelft WJ. (2004) Quality of primary care guidelines for acute low back pain. Spine. 29, E357-362.

Further information
- Iles V & Sutherland K. (2001) Managing Change in the NHS: A review for healthcare managers, professionals and researchers: National Co-ordinating Centre for NHS Service Delivery and Organisation R&D.
- NHS. (1999) NHS Centre for Reviews and Dissemination: Getting evidence into practice. Effective Health Care 5.
- Cochrane Effective Practice and Organisation of Care Group. **http://www.epoc.cochrane.org/en/index.html and http://www.unc.edu/depts/rsc/funk/barrier1.html**

1.15 Using evidence in practice
Bernadette Henderson

Professional knowledge ~ evidence-based practice ~ sources of information ~ how relevant is the evidence to my everyday practice ~ how valid is the evidence? ~ how much time do I have? ~ closing the evidence/practice gap

Introduction

Evidence-based practice (EBP) is an approach to healthcare wherein health professionals use the best evidence possible, i.e. the most appropriate information available, to make clinical decisions for individual patients. EBP values, enhances and builds on clinical expertise, knowledge of disease mechanisms, and pathophysiology. It involves complex and conscientious decision making based not only on the available evidence but also on patient characteristics, situations and preferences. It recognises that healthcare is individualised and ever changing and involves uncertainties and probabilities. Ultimately EBP is the formalisation of the care process that the best clinicians have practised for generations. (McKibbon, 1998).

Put more simply, *'Evidence based clinical practice is an approach to decision making in which the clinician uses the best evidence available, in consultation with the patient, to decide upon the option which suits that patient best'* (Gray, 1997).

Many different types of knowledge inform clinical decisions and practice. Every therapeutic encounter is unique and as such requires healthcare practitioners to select the most relevant and appropriate knowledge for that particular individual and situation. Take a moment and reflect on the last patient you treated. What did you do? Why did you choose one treatment rather than another? What were your decisions based upon? What particular types of knowledge guided your practice?... Difficult isn't it?

Professional knowledge

There are different types of professional knowledge, including propositional knowledge and personal knowledge.

Propositional knowledge is research based and develops theories to explain events and predict outcomes. It is included in educational programmes, examinations and courses and undergoes quality control by academics, educationalists and editors, and through peer review and debate. Propositional knowledge is explicit in that it can be fully and clearly expressed or demonstrated. It is processed consciously. Propositional knowledge includes basic sciences, applied science and technical skills.

Personal knowledge is the complex cognitive store each individual clinician brings to a therapeutic encounter that allows them to think, reason and perform. It includes personalised propositional knowledge, experiential knowledge and personal knowledge of the particular patient and of oneself. Skill, competency and expertise are a part of this knowledge. Personal knowledge can be explicit where conscious intellectual activities such as thinking, reasoning, remembering and imagining can be expressed or tacit where the thinking behind decisions and actions cannot be openly expressed or explained. The different types of knowledge are interconnected. Professional practice knowledge encompasses a complete appreciation of the specialised knowledge base and the ability to know how and when to apply this knowledge through past experience and codes of professional conduct (Eraut, 1985).

Professional knowledge (Eraut, 1992) includes:

Propositional knowledge ('knowing that') including academic knowledge and ideas derived from other professionals.

Process knowledge ('knowing how') including skilled action and deliberative analysis in decision making, problem solving and planning.

Personal knowledge including experiences, personal theories and memories.

Ethical principles or socialisation into the professional approach, including gaining a sense of professional identity.

Evidence-based practice

Evidence-based practice involves systematically finding, appraising and acting on evidence of effectiveness. We all intend our clinical practice to be informed by the best available evidence. However, with the overwhelming, ever-increasing volume and accessibility of health-related information available to healthcare practitioners, transferring evidence into practice is a very real problem. A number of complicated

1.15

questions need to be considered by clinicians in order to translate what we know into what we do.
- What do we believe is reliable and relevant evidence in any particular situation?
- Where do we access timely, trustworthy information?
- How do we incorporate and demonstrate it in practice?

Many problems in clinical practice cannot be resolved by applying exclusively propositional knowledge to make objective judgments. Day to day problems faced by clinicians are often unique and frequently require experience, intuition and creativity to be used in making a decision. The ideal situation is to have informed clinical decisions, based on reliable and relevant information about the risks, benefits and costs of the available alternatives, applied in our daily practice. How, then, to attempt to sort through the complex and sometimes inconsistent array of evidence available, in order for the clinician and the patient to decide which interventions are appropriate for their care.

Sources of information

There are a variety of sources of information available:
- Text books.
- Original studies in journals.
- Nationally and internationally produced pre-appraised evidence.
- National and local clinical guidelines.
- National and local experts.
- Colleagues.

All sources have their own strengths and weaknesses, but three interacting attributes have been proposed in assessing the usefulness of information (MeReC Briefing, 2004).

$$\text{Usefulness of information} = \frac{\text{relevance} \times \text{validity}}{\text{time to locate and interpret}}$$

How relevant is the evidence to my everyday practice?

Consider how applicable the evidence is to everyday practice. Judge the relevance of the information in the light of your specific practice question. Using the COFF acronym can help you decide on relevance (Maskrey et al, 2005):

C – does the article require me to change my practice?
O – are the outcomes measured going to make my patients either live longer or live better.
F – is the intervention feasible to do in my practice.
F – do I see patients frequently who have the condition looked at in the paper.

If 'no' is the answer to any of these questions, then the information is unlikely to be useful.

How valid is the evidence?

Sackett et al (2000) introduced a hierarchy which categorises evidence in order of validity from strongest to weakest. This placed systematic reviews of randomised controlled trials (RCTs) as the strongest level of evidence (see Table 1).

TABLE 1
Levels of evidence for interventions

Level of evidence	Type of study
1a	Systematic reviews of randomised controlled trials (RCTs)
1b	Individual RCTs with narrow confidence interval
2a	Systematic reviews of cohort studies
2b	Individual cohort studies and low-quality RCTs
3a	Systematic reviews of case-controlled studies
3b	Case-controlled studies
4	Case series and poor-quality cohort and case-control studies
5	Expert opinion

Adapted from Sackett et al (2000).

How close to the truth is this information, can I trust this evidence? This is an important question for all practitioners to ask. Critical appraisal assesses the validity of primary sources of evidence and is an essential part of evidence-based practice. User-friendly

1.15

guides and worksheets to facilitate critical appraisal are easily available with a computer key stroke (see Table 2 for examples).

TABLE 2
Critical appraisal guidelines, worksheets and weblinks

Bandolier	www.jr2.ox.ac.uk/bandolier
Public Health Resource Unit	www.phru.nhs.uk/Pages/PHD/resources.htm
Centre for Evidence Based Medicine	www.cebm.net/?o=1023
Scottish Intercollegiate Guidelines Network	http://www.sign.ac.uk/guidelines/fulltext/50/annexc.html
Physiotherapy Evidence Database	http://www.pedro.fhs.usyd.edu.au/

How much time do I have?

You need to consider the time it will take to locate and accurately interpret information. There is a presumption that clinicians can regularly critically appraise clinical papers to inform their practice. Conscientious critical appraisal is difficult, time consuming and often not practical for busy healthcare professionals. It is often preferable to use pre-appraised summaries of evidence and guidance from reliable sources, where the task of critical appraisal has already been completed, in preference to primary sources (see Table 3 for examples). These sources use rigorous methods and the most robust evidence. There is no need to assess the validity of the information as this has already been performed.

Nationally and internationally produced practice guidelines provide recommendations based on research evidence. Consensus by experts is incorporated into guideline development when evidence is lacking. Using available high quality pre-appraised evidence and guidelines allows clinicians time to consider and discuss the implications on their practice and to be able to apply valid evidence to the benefit of patients. Alternatively primary sources of evidence using literature searches can be used in specific cases as long as the information is viewed in the context of the wider evidence base.

TABLE 3
Sources of pre-appraised summaries of evidence and guidance with weblinks

Bandolier	www.jr2.ox.ac.uk/bandolier
Cochrane Library	www.cochrane.org/
National Institute for Clinical Excellence	http://www.nice.org.uk/
Centre for Evidence Based Medicine at Oxford	www.cebm.net/?o=1123
Scottish Intercollegiate Guidelines Network	http://www.sign.ac.uk/guidelines/http://www.sign.ac.uk/guidelines/index.html
Physiotherapy Evidence Database	http://www.pedro.fhs.usyd.edu.au/
Up-to-Date	http://www.uptodate.com/)

Closing the evidence/practice gap

The classic steps involved in evidence-based practice are:
1 A clinical question or problem arises out of the care of a patient.
2 Construct a well defined clinical question from the case.
3 Decide on how much time you have available to gather evidence, select the most appropriate sources to explore.
4 Conduct a search using the most appropriate resources.
5 Appraise that evidence for its validity (that is closeness to the truth) and relevance (that is applicability in clinical practice).
6 Integrate that evidence with clinical practice and patient preferences and apply it to practice.
7 Evaluate your performance with the patient.

However, it is often difficult to address the numerous and diverse questions that arise in clinical practice using this process. A variety of different methods can be used to ensure that evidence is incorporated into clinical practice.

1.15

Continuous professional development (CPD)
CPD provides a framework for linking evidence with practice. Formally identifying sources of knowledge and evidence, critically reflecting on that evidence and describing how practice is influenced clarifies and formalises the link. CPD offers the opportunity to plan, act, record and review knowledge and its impact on practice.

Journal clubs
Journal clubs can fulfil a number of functions: keeping up with literature, promoting evidence-based practice, demonstrating continuous professional development and learning critical appraisal skills. It is important to have one person who takes responsibility for the club.

Peer discussion
Results from practitioner research should be shared and collaborative reflection encouraged. Question practice: create a culture where you incessantly question yourself and those around you. Constantly exchange opinion, expertise and information.

Supervision
Observation of and reflection on practice by peers and senior staff, including peers from other specialties and healthcare professions, will encourage knowledge and skills transfer.

Presentations
Regularly present case study reviews of both common and unique cases. Evaluate and discuss outcomes from interventions.

Clinical guidelines
If national guidelines are not available, produce your own locally. Organise interested others, review the relevant literature, obtain expert opinion, discuss your own current practice and develop a guideline.

IT skills
Easily accessible computers and computer searching skills are necessary for evidence to be available instantaneously.

Knowledge brokers
Dialogue between researchers and practitioners about how to put research findings into practice is rare. A knowledge broker is a person who facilitates the creation, sharing and use of knowledge in an organisation.

Attributes and skills of a knowledge broker
- Entrepreneurial (networking, problem-solving, innovating).
- Trusted and credible.
- Clear communicator.
- Understands the cultures of both the research and decision-making environments.
- Able to find and assess relevant research in a variety of formats.
- Facilitates, mediates and negotiates.
- Understands the principles of adult learning.

The development of a knowledge broker in therapy services or clinical directorates would enable theoretical and practical knowledge transfer and help narrow the gap between what we know and what we do.

Reference list
- Eraut, M. (1985) Knowledge creation and knowledge use in professional contexts. Studies in Higher Education, 10(2),117-133.

- Eraut, M. (1992) Developing the knowledge base: a process perspective on professional education. In Learning to Effect ed Barnett, R, pp 98-118. Open University Press, Buckingham, UK and the Society for Research into Higher Education.

- Gray, JAM. (1997) Evidence-based healthcare: how to make health policy and management decisions. Churchill Livingstone, London.

- Maskrey N, Peglar S, Underhill J. (2005) Working smarter with information [eLetter]. Rapid response to BMJ 2005;331:352. Available from: **http//bmj.bmjjournals.com/cgi/eletters/331/7512/352-b**

- McKibbon KA (1998). Evidence-based practice. Bulletin of the Medical Library Association 86 (3): 396-401.

- MeReC Briefing (2004). Using evidence to guide practice. Issue number 30. Available from: **http://www.npc.co.uk/MeReC_Briefings/briefing2004.htm**

- Sackett DL, Straus SE, Richardson WS, Rosenberg W and Haynes B.R. (2000) Evidence-based Medicine: How to Practice and Teach EBM. 2nd edn. Churchill Livingstone Inc, Edinburgh, Scotland.

1.16 Creating and sustaining supportive environments for research
Lisa Roberts and Stuart Fraser

Increasing scholarly output ~ getting started: what support is needed? ~ sustaining a research culture ~ the clinician's perspective ~ next steps

When clinicians have key research questions and academics have scholarly experience and contacts, together they can be a formidable team. If every physiotherapy department had an objective to increase its scholarly output, this would greatly strengthen the evidence base and status of the profession. This chapter provides some practical suggestions of how this vision can become a reality, based on the experience of one NHS physiotherapy department.

Increasing scholarly output

In September 2004, a lecturer from the School of Health Professions and Rehabilitation Sciences at the University of Southampton was seconded for nine hours per week to Southampton University Hospitals trust over a three-year period. The aim of this role, funded by the trust, was to facilitate scholarly activity across the physiotherapy service, by supporting clinicians to:
- Complete service evaluations.
- Undertake audits.
- Register for higher degrees.
- Deliver poster and platform presentations at local/national/international conferences.
- Submit papers for publication to peer-reviewed journals.
- Submit grant applications.
- Build links with the Research & Development Support Unit (RDSU), academic community and National Physiotherapy Research Network (NPRN) local hub.

The most important criterion for the clinicians was enthusiasm, since 'Nothing great was ever achieved without enthusiasm' (Ralph Waldo Emerson [1803–1882]). The first step in getting the process started was to identify clinicians to nurture who were already engaged in any of the above activities, or who were planning to within the next year. To help identify these staff, a questionnaire was developed (freely available by contacting the first author: L.C.Roberts@soton.ac.uk) and given to every member of staff from technical instructor to manager. The aims of the questionnaire were to:
- Determine the status of scholarly activity that already existed in the department.
- Identify the key clinicians to nurture.
- Establish the help that staff perceived they needed to deliver their scholarly outputs.

Getting started – what support is needed?

From the questionnaire results, clinicians who expressed interest in any of these areas met with the research mentor to develop an action plan for the resources and support they needed, together with the timescale and milestones for completion.

Having identified the key clinicians, the next initiative involved forming peer support groups of 4–6 clinicians who met every 3–4 weeks over lunchtime, as staff perceived this was a good time to stand back from clinical work and legitimately pause to think. At these meetings, members outlined their activities, reported on progress and used the skills and experiences of the group to help overcome barriers. A strength of the group structure was that the physiotherapists came from a range of clinical fields. Each group was set up with a timeline for supporting members until they had fulfilled their ambitions; the groups were not set up to last indefinitely.

Alongside the peer groups, a range of additional support was offered, including:
- Helping access appropriate research courses offered by the RDSU and externally.
- Reviewing and providing feedback on:
  - Abstracts for conferences
  - Grant applications
  - Thesis chapters
  - Reports
  - Drafts of papers
  - Travel award applications.
- Guidance for producing posters.
- An environment of 'critical friends' for practising oral presentations.
- Lobbying the Directorate to purchase the software SPSS (The Statistical Package for the Social Sciences).
- Encouraging membership of external networks, guideline development groups and so on.
- Circulating information of interest on courses, seminars, research jobs and sources of potential funding.

Uptake of this support and the pace of delivery were determined by the clinicians as they integrated the scholarly activities into their working lives. They negotiated time away from the clinical coal-face with varying degrees of success and this significantly affected their outputs.

1.16

The Southampton team was on a mission – to create a research culture within the physiotherapy department. Many clinicians view research as a bit like going to the dentist: we know it's good for us, it's likely to hurt a bit and it's definitely something that everyone else should do! This culture needs to change.

Sustaining a research culture

- Research is relevant to all levels of clinicians
- Dedicated time at work is needed to undertake scholarly activity
- Celebrate your department's scholarly successes

Research is not just for those who aspire to be consultants or educators; it cannot be left to a handful of physiotherapists within the academic community. To ensure that research has direct clinical relevance, who better to get involved than the clinicians directly involved in patient care?

In this example, staff were supported (from technical instructor grade through to band 8 superintendents and clinical specialists) wherever they were in their research journey. One of the most important groups to target were the clinicians who had completed a Masters degree and had not disseminated the findings at national or international level. All too often, the end goal had been successful completion of the thesis and graduation, after which staff had then 'run out of steam' when it came to disseminating their work. All offers of help for staff at this level were particularly well received.

Developing a research culture is however, not just about the attitudes and abilities of the clinical staff; they will require practical support from managers, such as dedicated time at work to undertake scholarly activity. This remains a major barrier within the NHS and needs to be adequately resourced to ensure that research is not perceived as some sort of 'hobby', with which staff engage in their own time. If they are expected to undertake this work as part of their Agenda for Change remit, time needs to be protected to enable this to happen, just as it would for clinical requirements. As staff got underway on their individual projects, scholarly successes were celebrated within sections and at departmental meetings. This raised the profile of these activities and already the culture was starting to change as some clinicians were on the road to research.

1.16

The clinician's perspective: Stuart's story

Sitting on a stage at the World Confederation for Physical Therapy conference in Vancouver, looking at approximately 300 other therapists, waiting to hear my presentation, I couldn't help wondering 'How on earth did I get here?'

Eighteen months earlier, I found myself saying I wanted to do something more challenging. Should I do an MSc, clinical doctorate or a smaller piece of research? I thought I'd put a toe in the water and start with a literature review. I already had a topic relating to my clinical practice and, as I thought, a simple question: 'What was cauda equina syndrome?'

With the help of a research mentor, I got through the initially daunting task of conducting a literature search. After accessing a vast number of articles, two colleagues helped review them and we developed a framework to structure the data. Regular meetings at this stage were vital to ensure that all articles were reviewed consistently.

It quickly became apparent that my 'simple' research was turning into an epic task: the framework had ballooned from a few pages to 25! I felt like I was sinking and it was hard to remain enthusiastic. Ongoing advice and encouragement became a life-raft however, and allowed the data to be processed in smaller, more manageable pieces.

It also dawned on me that this work was producing unexpected findings as there was little consistency in the definition and clinical presentation of cauda equina syndrome. Fuelled by this revelation and newfound belief in my work, I was encouraged to share the findings with other clinicians and so presented them at a national, inter-professional spinal conference. By now, I was certainly feeling more challenged! This work was well received, giving me a new burst of energy. I further developed the framework and submitted an abstract to the world conference. Hearing it had been accepted was a fantastic feeling – my 'simple' literature review was now going to an international audience and I was off to Canada!

So what has the research experience taught me? As a clinician it's easy to find a research question in an aspect of your work that you enjoy. Even a small piece of research can at times appear the size of a mountain, so mentoring and teamwork along with protected time are essential. When you are steering in uncharted waters, you may encounter some rough seas. Undertaking research will however, challenge you, change your clinical practice and open up new horizons. Keep believing in what you are doing and there can be great rewards at the end of the research rainbow!

Next steps

You too could undertake a research journey. If you have a topic, either from a BSc/MSc assignment or your current clinical practice; and the enthusiasm to turn it into a paper or presentation our top tips are:
- Don't go it alone: Team up with colleagues who have some experience of presenting and publishing.
- Make contact with your local RDSU and NPRN hub.
- Work out how you are going to protect time in your schedule to make it happen.
- Plan a strategy of actions and identify the resources you will need. Remember, asking for help is a strength, not a weakness.
- Talk to your managers about possibilities for peer support groups, mentoring opportunities and protected time. You never know what this may lead to.
- Be prepared to step outside your comfort zone. This step could change the way you practise and think, and inspire others to ground their practice in evidence.
- Go for it! This could open the door into a whole new world for you. As Albert Einstein said: 'In the middle of difficulty lies opportunity.' Good luck!

Mentorship: an overview 1.17
Claudia Fellmer

Definition of mentoring ~ mentoring functions ~ types of mentoring relationships ~ key recommendations

Definition

Mentoring is a relationship in which a person with advanced experience (the mentor), through encouragement and guidance, invests time, know-how and effort in increasing and improving another person's (the mentee's) knowledge and skills, and consequently their professional and personal growth (Kram, 1983; Fagenson-Eland et al, 2005).

It should be a mutual relationship in which the mentor also benefits from personal and professional growth, and from the satisfaction of challenging and making a difference to someone else's development (Clutterbuck, 2004).

The third, often less noticeable, stakeholder taking an interest in successful mentoring, is the organisation. Mentoring relationships which involve individuals in different departments or organisations can provide useful networking opportunities, and lead to increased creativity due to shared and better utilised knowledge. Knowledge sharing can vastly improve the way an organisation is run, and increase organisational effectiveness (Burke et al, 1993; Ragins, 1999).

> The term mentor is said to originate in Greek legend, where Ulysses entrusted the education of his son Telemachus to the wise counsellor Mentor (actually the Goddess Athena in disguise) for the duration of his voyage.

Mentoring functions

Mentoring is generally an integrated approach, comprising a number of functions. Traditionally these have been categorised into career and psychological functions: the former enabling mentees to gain organisational exposure and learn how to achieve promotions; the latter providing role modelling and counselling 'resulting in an increased sense of competence, effectiveness and self-worth' (Fowler and O'Gorman, 2005). However, recent findings indicate that this clear-cut division between different types of mentoring function cannot be maintained.

Fowler and O'Gorman (2005) identified eight distinct functions of mentoring. Their work reassessed previous findings (for example the pioneering work by Kram 1980 and 1985; and the work by Ragins (1990) and McFarlin (1990) and they conducted their own mixed methods study. The results revealed a more convincing analysis than the traditional view that there were only two main functions, and also showed that mentees and mentors share similar perceptions about mentoring functions. (See Figure 1 below).

FIGURE 1

Personal and emotional guidance	involves psychological counselling, acceptance and confirmation
Coaching	develops ideas, expands knowledge into a particular direction and is fairly directive (for example mentor describes own experience)
Advocacy	the mentor promotes the mentee within networks and the organisational hierarchy (though only with a marginal degree of protection as the current organisational climate does not perceive this as guidance beneficial to the mentee)
Career development facilitation	career guidance and advice on options with limited conflict of interest (as mentor is not the line manager)
Role modelling	the attitudes, values and behaviour of the mentor provide a standard to emulate
Strategies and systems advice	sharing understanding and knowledge of informal and organisational-political processes, provide access to information mostly available through higher-level members of the organisation
Learning facilitation	provides feedback to the mentee after a particular task, reflection on experience (meta-skills of self-reflection)
Friendship	social support network

Facilitating learning

In the clinical and academic environment most people have a lot of experience and expertise in a few specific areas. However, as soon as they cross the boundaries to a new topic, or new methodology, they have little knowledge. They assume the paradoxical status of expert 'novices'.

The best way forward for mentors is to provide mentees with what can be called maieutic support: this is where mentors aim not to provide the solutions, but rather to help their mentees to learn how to get to the solution. The maieutic method was first described by ancient Greek scholar Socrates to define a process by which a mentor assists a mentee to become fully conscious of ideas already latent in the mind (cf. online Oxford English Dictionary). The mentor should therefore strive to be non-directive and yet stretching in her/his guidance.

Overarching mentoring styles
A matrix of overarching mentoring functions can be developed along the two dimensions, 'who is in charge?' (from directive to non-directive) and 'what does the individual need?' (from stretching/challenging to nurturing). From these dimensions the four basic styles of helping emerge: coaching, guiding, counselling and networking.

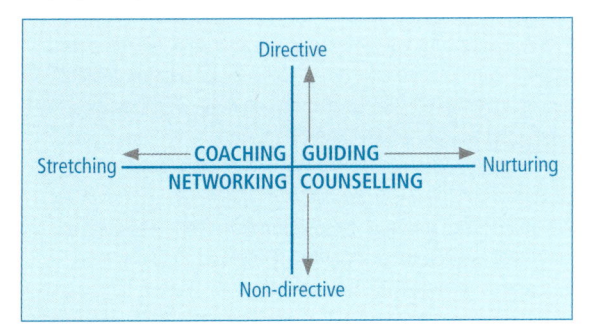

```
                    Directive
                       ▲
                       │
         ┌─── COACHING │ GUIDING ───┐
Stretching            │             Nurturing
         └─── NETWORKING│ COUNSELLING┘
                       │
                       ▼
                  Non-directive
```

(Clutterbuck, 2004)

Different styles in different environments
There are significant cultural differences in relation to mentoring. Clutterbuck (2004) distinguishes 'developmental mentoring' from 'sponsoring mentoring'. The former emphasises 'empowerment and personal accountability' for the mentee, and an even balance of all four styles of mentoring. Sponsoring mentoring, on the other hand, prioritises the 'effective use of power and influence' by the mentor, predominately through guidance and counselling. Preferences for one style or the other relate both to the wider culture (for example the UK shows a preference towards developmental mentoring compared to the USA) and the internal organisational environment (strongly hierarchical structures favour sponsoring styles).

The developmental-sponsoring balance is also determined by the status of the individual relationship, and will change over time.

Types of mentoring relationships

Informal versus formal systems

The manner in which mentoring relationships are established and conducted is referred to as formal or informal. Formal relationships emerge when an organisation is attempting to establish them by bringing mentors and mentees together systematically. The criteria for this tend to be based on mentor expertise, mentee needs, a system of guidelines and rules and also, often, on a set of organisational expectations (outcomes).

By contrast, informal relationships are initiated by individuals and are based on mutual liking and rapport before they focus on areas of expertise. Here, meetings take place as and when required by the partners within the mentoring relationship. It is also suggested that the quality (or effectiveness) of the informal mentoring relationship is higher: the mentoring partners' personalities and related cognitive styles may be a better match because they have not been assigned to each other (Armstrong et al., 2002; Ragins and Cotton, 1999). There are a number of benefits and disadvantages to formally and informally established mentoring relationships (see Figure 2) (Niehoff, 2006).

Several studies assessing the benefits of informal versus formal mentoring suggest a significant advantage for informal mentoring relationships. However, organisations wishing to establish a mentoring scheme may have to take the formal route for a number of years. Once a mentoring culture has developed, this may allow a transition to more informal routes.

Multiple mentors and peer mentoring

Traditionally the mentoring relationship is defined as a dyad: a mentee has one mentor, replicating a student-teacher relationship. However, the more recent emphasis on networks has led to studies defining mentoring in terms of peers: mentees support one another, and mentors often support other mentors in selected areas of expertise. Furthermore, mentees can have other mentors alongside their primary mentor across the hierarchical levels, such as peers, subordinates or other superiors, both within and outside the organisation. This idea of the network also recognises the fact that mentoring relationships will shift and change over time, and are by no means set in stone.

1.17

FIGURE 2
Informal v formal mentoring

Informal mentoring	Formal mentoring
Volitional, develops spontaneously	Develops with organisational assistance/intervention (voluntary assignment possible)
Participants have choice of selection (mutual identification)	Participants may have some choice in selection
Interpersonal comfort: personality allowed to an influence on selection, for example 'a chemistry that sparks'	Personality may be considered, but if so have by a third party. Allocation through a third party is easier for people new to an organisation (for example in an induction period), as they lack the inside knowledge and potential mentors do not know them yet
Often no structured guidelines	Organisation provides guidelines and training (clearer understanding of what is expected and how to achieve these goals)
Develop on basis of perceived competence of mentor and perceived performance potential of mentee ('diamond in the rough')	Assigned on expertise as perceived by organisation/a co-ordinator or on basis of application forms
Goals and expectations evolve over time to adapt to specific needs	Goals specified at start positive aspects of having an external 'force' which 'disciplines' adherence to self-set goals
Meet when needed and desired	Meetings scheduled and time allotted
Carry no explicit rewards or sanctions	Explicit rewards or sanctions
Long in duration, on average 3–6 years	Short in duration on average 6 months to 1 year
Mentees tend to receive more career development support (sponsoring, coaching, exposure, challenging assignments, protection)	
Higher occurrence of psychosocial functions (for example friendship, social support, role modelling, acceptance)	
Mentees experience greater satisfaction with their mentors	

(Ragins and Cotton 1999; Niehoff 2006)

Key recommendations

Organisational level
- organisations keen to enhance their effectiveness should foster a mentoring culture.
- develop guidelines, preferably semi-formal, to support mentees and mentors.
- facilitate mentoring training.
- introduce a mentoring culture through a period of primarily formal processes and then allow transfer to informal.
- encourage peer and multiple relationships.
- have process/contact person if things go wrong.

Relationship level
- each relationship sets its own rules regarding the level of formality (frequency, style of meetings, outputs) in correspondence with the organisational guidelines.
- mentees are given a choice of mentor.
- to avoid a conflict of interests, a mentor must not be the line manager of the mentee.
- mentoring relationships are flexible and not permanent.
- consider use of mentors external to the organisation.

Reference list
- Allen TD and Poteet ML (1999) 'Developing effective mentoring relationships: Strategies from the mentor's viewpoint', Career Development Quarterly, vol. 48, pp.59-73; referenced in Fowler and O'Gorman (2005).
- Armstrong SJ, Allinson CW and HayesJ. (2002), 'Formal mentoring systems: an examination of the effects of mentor/protégé cognitive styles on the mentoring process', Journal of Management Studies, vol. 39, no. 8, pp.1111-37.
- Burke RJ, McKeen CA and McKeena C. (1993), 'Correlates of mentoring in organizations: The mentor's perspective', Psychological Reports, vol. 72, pp.883-96.
- Clutterbuck D. (2004), Everyone needs a mentor: Fostering talent in your organisation, 4th edition, London: Chartered Institute of Personnel and Career Development.
- Fagenson-Eland, EA, Baugh SG and Lankau MJ. (2005), 'Seeing eye to eye: A dyadic investigation into the effect of relational demography on perceptions of mentoring activities', Career Development International, vol. 10, no. 6/7, pp.460-77.
- Fowler JL and O'Gorman JG. (2005), 'Mentoring functions: A contemporary view of the perceptions of mentees and mentors', British Journal of Management, vol. 16, pp.51-7.

1.17

- Kram KE. (1980), Mentoring at work: Developmental relationships in managerial career, unpublished PhD thesis Yale University, New Haven, USA.
- Kram KE. (1985), Mentoring at work: Developmental relationships in organizational life, Scott, Foresman, Glenview, IL, USA.
- Megginson D and Clutterbuck D. (2006), 'Creating a coaching culture', Industrial and Commercial Training, vol. 38, no. 5, pp.232-37.
- Niehoff BP. (2006), 'Personality predictors of participation as a mentor', Career Development International, vol. 11, no. 4, pp.321-333.
- Ragins BR. (1999), 'Where do we go from here and how do we get there? Methodological issues in conducting research on diversity and mentoring relationships', in: Murrell AJ, Crosby FJ and Ely RJ. (eds.), Mentoring Dilemmas: Developmental relationships within multicultural organizations, pp.227-47, Mahwah, NJ, USA: Erlbaum; referenced in Fowler and O'Gorman (2005).
- Ragins BR and Cotton JL. (1999), 'Mentor functions and outcomes: A comparison of men and women in formal and informal mentoring relationships', Journal of Applied Psychology, vol. 84, no. 4, pp.529-550.
- Ragins BR and McFarlin. (1990) Perceptions of mentor roles in cross-gender mentoring relationships. Journal of Vocational Behaviour vol. 37: 321-339.

Further information
- Scheck McAlearney A. (2005), 'Exploring mentoring and leadership development in health care organizations', Career Development International, vol. 10, no. 6/7, pp.493-511.

1.18 Mentorship schemes: an example
Adam Garrow

Introduction ~ the Training and Mentorship (TRAM) scheme ~ TRAM applicants ~ modifications of TRAM ~ further information

Health Research and Development North West's Training and Mentorship scheme (TRAM): an introduction

In the previous section, the approach to mentoring as an activity conducted by a person (the mentor) for another person (the mentee) was discussed. It is generally agreed that the objective of the mentoring process is to promote individual development with the help of the experience, knowledge and advice of the designated mentor. It is also acknowledged that mentoring is not a 'one-off' event. Individuals will often require different kinds of mentoring from different people at key stages of their career as a researcher, particularly when reviewing their career options.

It is also important that any NHS scheme is both appropriate to meet the needs of individuals, and compatible with the overall aims and objectives of the local healthcare institution and ultimately the Department of Health.

This section presents an outline of an innovative mentorship scheme, and shows how the scheme has been adapted to meet the requirements of the ever changing NHS. It may be a useful example on which other mentoring schemes can be modelled.

There are a number of examples of generic mentoring schemes in the NHS, including the Get a Guru scheme in the East Midlands (NHS, 2007) and the North West Mentoring Scheme (Greater Manchester Strategic Health Authority, 2005). Although there is already a mentoring scheme to guide and support medically-qualified researchers who are interested in developing their research leadership potential (Academy of Medical Sciences, 2008), similar schemes are not yet widely available to other healthcare professions.

To address this need, Health Research and Development North West (R&D NoW) introduced a competitive research Training and Mentorship (TRAM) scheme.

R&D NoW is a partnership between the universities of Lancaster, Liverpool and Salford and a member of the national network of Research and Development Support Units (RDSUs) funded by the Department of Health (DH). RDSUs are being replaced by the Research Design Services (RDS) (NHS NIHR, 2008) and will have an important new role in supporting applications for research funding, such as the Research for Patient Benefit Scheme (RfPB) (NHS NIHR, 2007), as well as other external funding bids.

The Training and Mentorship (TRAM) Scheme

On entering the scheme, each of the TRAM Fellows have a meeting with one of the Directors at Health R&D NoW, all of whom are lead researchers at the three host universities. During this meeting, the Fellows are able to discuss their general aims and objectives, and their training and mentoring needs. Since the scheme was designed to attract research-active health care professionals, the TRAM Fellows usually have a good idea about who they would like as a mentor. A key role of the R&D NoW Director therefore involves ensuring the suitability of the proposed mentor, and arranging the first formal mentoring appointment between the mentor and mentee.

At this initial meeting, the mentor and mentee draw up an outline Personal Development Plan (PDP) for the Fellowship. The PDP is an opportunity for the TRAM Fellows to focus their ideas and document their specific training and mentoring needs. The PDP also provides a record of how the individual develops as a researcher within the scheme. Throughout the scheme the TRAM Fellows are also encouraged to provide feedback to Health R&D NoW, with comments and suggestions on how the scheme could be improved. In this way, the TRAM scheme attempts to address both individual needs, and the wider needs of the NHS.

TRAM applicants

The TRAM scheme has attracted applications from a wide variety of healthcare professional backgrounds, including physiotherapy, palliative care, dentistry and nursing. Not surprisingly, the individual training needs are equally varied, with the Fellows wishing to develop an expertise in qualitative and quantitative research methods, dissemination skills and the writing of grant proposals. Mentoring, however, is at the heart of the TRAM scheme, and the success of the scheme depends on the Fellows establishing a close and equal working relationship with their appointed mentors. There are many ways the TRAM Fellows benefit from the knowledge and expertise of their mentor. Some benefits, such as advising and directing the Fellows to the most appropriate training course, are obvious and measurable; others are less tangible, but equally important in helping the Fellows focus their research ambitions and plan their future research career. A good example of this is the opportunity to establish links with the Clinical Research Networks and develop and discuss research ideas with other healthcare professionals in the North West of England. In this way, rather than being considered as simply a year-long training award, the intention of the TRAM scheme is to provide the Fellows with a firm platform from which they can launch their future research career.

1.18

Modifications of TRAM to match new National Institute of Health Research (NIHR) objectives

Initially the TRAM scheme concentrated on methodological issues, where individual Fellows identified a specific need for qualitative or quantitative training. Another vitally important skill needed by healthcare researchers is the ability to develop high quality research proposals for external funding applications. Researchers writing their first application soon discover that preparing a funding bid is time consuming, complex, frustrating and if, after an enormous amount of effort the application is rejected, deeply disheartening. The National Institute of Health Research (NIHR) has introduced a great variety of funding initiatives. Some funding, such as the New and Emerging Applications of Technology (NEAT) awards and the programme grants for allied research (NHS NIHR, 2007) are for substantial amounts of money, and are probably more suited to applicants from established research groups or researchers familiar with the conduct of multiple centre studies. On the other hand, the Research for Patient Benefit Scheme (RfPB) (NHS NIHR, 2008) is likely to be more attractive to healthcare professionals of all disciplines. It is specifically designed to support research related to the everyday practice of health service staff and to have a demonstrable impact on users of the service. However, the national rejection rate in the first two calls was very high. Feedback from RfPB commissioning panels suggested that, although many of the applications contained excellent ideas with potential for real patient benefit, many of the projects could not be funded because of important methodological flaws. RfPB panels also commented that proposals could have been strengthened by specialist advice and guidance. This will be part of the new role of the Research Design Services when they become fully operational in October 2008, and is also available from NPRN hubs.

To ensure compatibility with the new RDS brief, Health RDS NoW now provides support and mentoring to all local researchers to help them prepare proposals for RfPB and other national, peer-reviewed funding competitions in health or social care research. Instead of general research methods training, the emphasis will now concentrate on specific components of an application such as medical ethics, user involvement and the principles of full economic costing. At the heart of the new organisation in the North West, is a team of Senior Research Advisers (SRAs) who are established NHS or academic researchers with a successful record of securing awards through the NIHR, and other external funding sources. Researchers preparing bids can now obtain general advice about the funding schemes and the application process through their local Research Design Service office and specialist advice from the Senior Research Advisers. If necessary, this can be supplemented by a team of Research Design Advisers for focused methodological and statistical advice. The ultimate aim of the process is to improve the quality of grant applications and, therefore, increase the chances of success. For healthcare professionals who do not yet have the necessary experience to be a Principal Investigator, an important role of the RDS will be to pull together a project research team with the breadth and depth of experience required to submit a successful grant application. In this way, healthcare professionals will be able to develop a portfolio of projects while working alongside a team of experienced researchers and, through this experience, ultimately become Principal Investigators in their own right.

This supplementary section on mentoring provided an example of a mentoring scheme that brings together the ambitious aims and objectives of the NHS and the personal research aspirations of healthcare professionals. Since its inception, the scheme has needed to adapt to meet both the contractual obligations of the Research Design Services and the stated aim of the NHS. In the future, the NHS will require healthcare professionals across all disciplines to develop greater expertise in research. This will be supported in a variety of ways including, through a variety of competitively funded personal development opportunities administered through the NHS Research Capacity Development Programme (NHS NIHR, 2007).

Recognising that grant applications need to be of high quality to stand a good chance of success, the NIHR now provides healthcare professionals with the advice and support they need to put together well-designed applications to personal development schemes, as well as responsive mode funding schemes such as Research for Patient Benefit. Although this kind of targeted support was previously restricted to NHS researchers working in the North West of England, it is now becoming available nationally through the new Research Design Services although the way the service is delivered may vary from region to region.

Reference list
- The Academy of Medical Sciences. (2008) Mentoring Programme [online]. Available from **http://www.academicmedicine.ac.uk/mentoring/amsprog.aspx**
- Greater Manchester Strategic Health Authority. (2005). The North West Mentoring Scheme [online]. Available from **http://www.gmsha.nhs.uk/mentoring/index.html**
- The NHS Improvement Network – East Midlands. (2007). Get a Guru [online]. Available from **http://www.tin.nhs.uk/get-a-guru**
- NHS National Institute for Health Research. (2007). NIHR Calls and Proposals [online]. Available from **http://www.nihr-ccf.org.uk/site/callsproposals/default.cfm**
- NHS National Institute for Health Research. (2007). National Coordinating Centre for Research Capacity Development [online]. Available from **http://www.nccrcd.nhs.uk/**
- NHS National Institute for Health Research. (2008). The Research Design Services (RDS) [online] Available from **http://www.nihr-ccf.org.uk/site/programmes/rfpb/default.cfm**
- NHS National Institute for Health Research. (2008). The Research for Patient Benefit (RfPB) Programme [online]. Available from **http://www.nihr-ccf.org.uk/site/programmes/rfpb/default.cfm**

2.1 Developing a research career pathway
Gabrielle Rankin

Introduction ~ career frameworks and pathways ~ what you need to know about research jobs ~ combined roles ~ key research policies ~ choosing your research topic(s) ~ research training ~ mentors and networking

Introduction

Physiotherapy and the other AHPs are emergent professions with respect to academic development and research. Degrees were first awarded to British physiotherapists in 1979 and around that same time a couple of physiotherapists became the first to be awarded PhDs in subjects related to physiotherapy. It is only since September 1993 that physiotherapy has been an all degree entry profession in the UK. Research careers for AHPs are not yet well established but this is changing and clearer research pathways are starting to evolve.

In planning a research career you should understand the main career path options. These are mapped out in career frameworks. You need to know what a job entails and the requirements for different job roles. You should also be aware of the bigger picture – what is happening in the health and education sectors that may influence research career options.

Once you have considered where you want to go you can plan how to get there. Think about what research areas interest you and how you can build up your research experience and training. The best advice you can get is from those who have already developed a research career – a mentor and networking are invaluable.

Career frameworks and pathways

- Healthcare Framework
- Higher Education Framework
- Health and Education Framework

The main frameworks are for healthcare, higher education and combined pathways. In some sectors, for example, industry and private practice, research career pathways are less well defined.

Healthcare Framework
Skills for Health have developed a generic framework, the Career Framework for Health. A number of other more specific frameworks have been developed, including one for AHPs **www.skillsforhealth.org.uk**.

Key concepts to understand:
There are nine progressive levels within the framework with levels five to nine being relevant for qualified physiotherapists. It is important to note that framework levels do not directly correspond to the nine NHS pay bands (see below).

Job roles are described in terms of knowledge, skills and competences. These can be thought of as transferable currency and allow more flexible career options within healthcare.

Career pathways are being developed around care pathways and priority patient/user groups rather than clinical specialities or professions. An example of how research knowledge, skills and competences may be integrated into pathways is the Public Health Skills and Career Framework **www.phru.nhs.uk**.

Higher Education Framework
The Higher Education Framework Agreement for the Modernisation of Pay Structures is the national grading and pay framework for all staff working in higher education institutes. Within the Framework there are examples of career pathways for academic staff which all have five levels. In the research pathway the levels are broadly described as:

Level 1   Assist in research activity
Level 2   Carry out research as an individual or team member
Level 3   Conducting research programmes
Level 4   Leading research teams
Level 5   Development and overall management of research programmes

A national library of academic role profiles at each level has been developed to describe the demands and responsibilities of staff who have a research role or who have combined teaching and research roles **www.ucea.ac.uk**

Health and Education Framework
The Strategic Learning and Research Advisory Group (StLaR) was established by the Departments of Health and for Education and Skills and has looked at the human

2.1

resources (HR) issues faced by researchers and educators working in health and social care. Their HR plan addresses some of the problems of joint employment and also has exemplar career pathways **www.stlarhr.org.uk**

What you need to know about research jobs

- Job descriptions and person specifications
- Competences
- Agenda for Change (AfC)
- The Knowledge and Skills Framework (KSF)
- Qualifications
- Comparison of HEI and NHS pathways
- Job adverts

Job descriptions and person specifications
Every HEI research post will have a job description including main duties and responsibilities and a person specification including the required qualifications, training, knowledge, skills and experience.

NHS job descriptions are becoming more complex and require an understanding of competences, the KSF and AfC.

Competences
Competences describe the work *activities* that need to be carried out to achieve a particular purpose, the *quality standards* to which these activities need to be performed and the *knowledge and skills* needed to carry out these activities

Within the Career Framework for Health competences are nationally recognised and transferable across all sectors of healthcare – NHS, independent and voluntary. Groups or 'suites' of competences have been developed for different service areas and disciplines. There is a suite of 16 research and development (R&D) competences and it is useful to look at the description for each of these **www.skillsforhealth.org.uk**
Each competence is also linked to the Knowledge and Skills Framework (see below).

Agenda for Change (AfC)
This is the pay system for all NHS staff except doctors, dentists and most senior managers. National job profiles have been developed for clinical researchers, AHPs

(consultants) and for physiotherapists. Each profile has a title and pay banding. There are nine incremental pay bands from Band 1 to Band 9 with Band 8 having four ranges A–D. You will find it particularly helpful to look at the research profiles which have been published at Bands 6, 7, 8A and 8B-C-D **www.nhsemployers.org**

The Knowledge and Skills Framework (KSF)
The KSF is part of AfC and describes the knowledge and skills that healthcare practitioners apply in their roles. It also includes an annual system of review and development for staff which identifies learning and development needs and is the mechanism through which pay progression operates.

Each NHS post has a job description and a KSF post outline setting out how knowledge and skills should be applied in the role. A national library of profiles is available at **www.e-ksf.org**

Qualifications
It is not yet clear how the NHS Career Framework will link to educational qualifications. There is a knowledge, training and experience section in each AfC profile which indicates what qualifications are required. In relation to the HEI pathway levels, those working at level 1 would normally be undertaking a PhD and at level 2 would normally have a PhD or three years' research experience or an MSc and two years' research experience.

Job adverts
- Frontline and the CSP website advertise a relatively small number of research posts.
- National press – the Education Guardian (Tuesdays) and Times Higher Education Supplement.
- Internet – **www.jobs.ac.uk, www.jobs.nhs.uk, www.jobs.guardian.co.uk www.timeshighereducation.co.uk/jobs_home.asp**
- Website vacancy pages for specific trusts or HEIs.

Combined roles

- Lecturer
- Consultant posts
- Clinical academic posts
- Key issues

2.1

Lecturer
Lecturer posts offer combined teaching and research roles (see chapter 2.12). More recently, combined research, teaching and clinical posts have been developed.

Consultant posts
The consultant role consists of four inter-related core functions – expert practice; professional leadership and consultancy; education and professional development; practice and service development, research and evaluation. More details can be found in a CSP information paper: Physiotherapy Consultant (NHS): Role, Attributes and Guidance for Establishing Posts PA56 2002 **www.csp.org.uk**

Clinical academic posts
These are joint posts where a university, a trust or in some cases both are the employer. Lecturer practitioner posts combine teaching, clinical and research roles.

Currently there are relatively few posts which combine clinical and research roles but this is likely to change as increasingly, NHS research funding is awarded to Trust and HEI partnerships and especially when recommendations from the UKCRC nurses report are implemented for AHPs (see below).

Key issues
Clinical academic posts can be very attractive but there are a number of potential issues especially if you have two employers:

Combined roles
- Is the job description realistic?
- Is it clear what percentage of time should be devoted to each role and how it will be divided – is there any flexibility in this?
- Is time for different roles protected in any way?
- Will you have resources for training to develop knowledge and skills in each role?
- Are there adequate facilities and infrastructure to support you in all your roles?

Joint contracts
- Will you be employed by the NHS/HEI or both ?
- Permanent or fixed term contract? (fixed term more common with HEI employer).
- Grading and salary.
- Pension arrangements.
- Appraisal and staff development systems.
- Look at the StLaR HR plan (see above).

Key research policies

- NHS strategy.
- Department of Health.
- UK Clinical Research Collaboration (UKCRC) clinical academic careers.
- Higher Education Funding Councils.

Policy documents are daunting for most people but whatever career pathway you are considering, you are more likely to be successful with some political awareness. It helps to be familiar with government research strategies. Look at executive summaries for key messages and consider the potential implications for you and other AHP researchers. Each of the four UK countries have different policies which can differ significantly. Important websites for each country are given below. *Frontline*, the CSP website **www.csp.org.uk** and interactive website **www.interactivecsp.org.uk** and your NPRN hub will also alert you to major developments.

NHS strategy
Lord Darzi's review, *Our NHS, our future – the NHS Next Stage Review* will have a huge impact on the services that the NHS delivers. Although it primarily addresses the NHS in England it is likely that the other UK countries will implement recommendations within the report. The interim report was published in October 2007 and the final report published in July 2008.

What do you need to know?
- NHS priorities – you are not likely to get NHS research funding if your research areas do not align with these priorities **www.ournhs.nhs.uk**

Department of Health
Best Research for Best Health is the research strategy for England and led to the development of the National Institute for Health Research (NIHR).

What do you need to know?
- The NIHR website has information about all NHS research funding **www.nihr.ac.uk**
- Clinical research networks set up to support research studies and promote patient and public involvement in health research – Cancer, Dementias and Neurodegenerative diseases, Diabetes, Medicines for Children, Mental Health and

2.1

Stroke; Primary Care and Comprehensive Clinical Research Networks Research posts and training programmes are available through these networks **www.ukcrn.org.uk**
- The research capacity development programme – Research Training (PhD), Post-Doctoral, Career Development and Senior Research Fellowships **www.nccrcd.org.uk**
- For Northern Ireland, Scotland or Wales the relevant websites are **www.dhsspsni.gov.uk/ahp_research www.sehd.scot.nhs.uk/cso www.word.wales.gov.uk**

UKCRC clinical academic careers
Developing the best research professionals Qualified graduate nurses: recommendations for preparing and supporting clinical academic nurses of the future is a report that addresses training and career pathways for nurses combining clinical and academic roles.

What do you need to know?
- If you are considering a combined clinical academic career look at the recommendations in the report. It is likely that the recommendations will also be implemented and funded for AHPs in the near future **www.nccrcd.org.uk**

Higher Education Funding Councils
Each of the four UK countries has a Council which funds the research infrastructure in HEIs and the salaries of permanent academic staff. The quality of research in research departments of each HEI is regularly rated, currently through the research assessment exercises (RAE) but in the future using the Research Excellence Framework (REF). This determines how funding is allocated to each department.

What do you need to know?
- How will the quality of your research be assessed? **www.hefce.ac.uk/research** (England), **www.delni.gov.uk** (Nothern Ireland – follow links to further and higher education), **www.sfc.ac.uk** (Scotland), **www.hefcw.ac.uk** (Wales).
- How well has a specific research department done in previous RAEs? **www.rae.ac.uk**

Choosing your research topic(s)

If you have a clinical background you will probably want to undertake research which relates to your clinical interests especially if you are considering a career with combined roles.
However, bear in mind that research posts and funding are relatively scarce. You may need to think about applying for studentships or research posts in areas that are not

your first choice. If your research interests do not fall within the research priorities of the main research funders it will be much harder to find funding to pursue your research.

Look at the research themes in the HEIs, research centres and networks located in your area. It will be easier to access expertise and resources if your research fits within their programmes. If you have very specific and narrow research interests you may need to be prepared to move locations.

Above all, you need to feel inspired by the research projects you are involved in!

Research training

- Information on training.
- Funding.
- Training for research or combined roles.

Information on training
- Database of more than 500 post-qualifying programmes of interest to physiotherapists **www.csp.org.uk**
- CSP information papers:
  Registering for a research degree RES 04 October 2001 – this has tips about choosing the right university and department
  Master's Level Programmes Within Postqualifying Physiotherapy Education: SP Criteria and Expectations QA 03 2003
  Professional and taught doctorates CSP criteria and expectations QA 04 2005.
  www.csp.org.uk
- Databases of research degrees, short courses, workshops and conferences with specific AHP editions **www.rdlearning.org.uk**
- Websites of specific HEIs – what are their research themes and projects, how many research staff and doctoral students?

Funding
- Databases for Fellowships and Studentships, AHPs, funding from government, professional bodies and research councils **www.rdfunding.org.uk**

2.1

Training for research or combined roles

Before choosing a research degree programme it is important to consider the amount of research training provided and practical research undertaken especially in different doctoral programmes. Currently the eligibility criteria for some postdoctoral research fellowships stipulate that you must have a PhD rather than professional or taught doctorate. University websites may provide details about the structure and delivery of their programmes, also request their programme handbook. If possible, speak to someone currently undertaking the programme.

Mentors and networking

The different things you need to be aware of and consider in planning a career in healthcare research can be overwhelming.

Having access to a mentor is extremely useful. A mentor will support and assist you in your personal and professional development and provide career guidance. For more information see the CSP information paper Mentoring: an overview CSP35 2005 **www.csp.org.uk**

Mentoring can be formal or informal. Mentoring schemes are starting to be developed as part of research training programmes. If you do not have access to a formal mentoring scheme you may be able to get help from your local NPRN hub.

Networking will play an essential part in developing your career. Make use of any relevant research or clinical networks, including multidisciplinary and international networks. Conferences are a great way of making new contacts and most researchers are very happy to be emailed and to discuss their research.

Seize any opportunity to talk to others who have already embarked on a research career. Reading this book is a good starting point!

The new graduate's first steps into research 2.2
Suzanne McDonough and David Baxter

Using evidence to support practice ~ further research training ~ masters programmes ~ PhD training ~ making the right networks ~ pump priming funding ~ prioritise research

Once qualified, there are a variety of routes through which you can get involved in research, depending on your career aspirations. You may be interested at this stage in looking at the information compiled by the Department of Health (DH) via the Strategic Learning and Research (StLaR) Group, which describes different possible career routes in clinical and academic settings (see **www.stlarhr.org.uk** for more information).

Be proactive: use evidence to support practice

Remember that through your undergraduate training you already have the necessary skills in how to ask a research question, and to appraise the pertinent literature. You should take the opportunity to practise and refine these skills, perhaps through a formal literature review. Is there an aspect of your practice about which you are unsure: for example, is it clear that a certain treatment is effective, or how should you best administer the treatment? Use your training to look at the literature in order to try and answer such questions. At this stage is will be helpful to involve your colleagues in this process, for example:
- Offer to present your research question at an in-service training session or NPRN event. It may help you establish a network of colleagues with interests in this area, or help you refine your question.
- Speak to academic colleagues where you trained as an undergraduate.
- Present any findings from your review within your clinical setting; or
- If appropriate, consider presenting your findings at a suitable research conference [Physiotherapy Research Society (PRS), Rehabilitation and Therapy Research Society (RTRS), CSP congress].

By taking this type of approach, it will help you to realise whether you would like to get advanced training in reviewing the literature. At this stage, there is a range of options: you could apply to undertake a postgraduate course (for example, a Masters programme will usually incorporate teaching in advanced research skills); you could access training via the Cochrane library; or in Ireland (North and South) you can apply for a Cochrane Fellowship, which provides two years of funding to 'buy you out' of your clinical post for two days per week. This provides the necessary training to carry out a Cochrane review. In order to apply for a fellowship you must have an established link with a Cochrane group, plus university academic support (see the section on making networks below).

Other potential sources of funding include the CSP Physiotherapy Research Foundation (PRF). This specifically runs a scheme of funding for novice researchers; again, you need to have established a network before you apply for funding.

Further research training

The CSP keeps details of more than 500 postqualifying programmes of interest to physiotherapists. You can use the CSP's postqualifying programmes database to conduct an online search by geographic region or subject area (see: **http://www.csp.org.uk/director/careersandlearning/continuingprofessionaldevelopment/postqualifyingprogrammes.cfm**). This provides information on postgraduate certificates, diplomas and masters programmes.

Masters programmes
(for example, Masters of Clinical Research)

The Masters of Clinical Research was developed in response to the need for tailored postgraduate research education for physiotherapists and other professionals working in the health service **(http://prospectus.ulster.ac.uk/course/?id=4410)**. The Northern Ireland (NI) R&D office provides bursaries (includes costs for fees and research expenses) for healthcare professionals who wish to apply for this course, if they are working in the health service in Northern Ireland. A key module on this course is on clinical research techniques, the outcome of which is the submission of a research proposal. This module is taken partly by distance (e-learning) and partly by university attendance, and provides a grounding for anyone in need of expert guidance on writing a research proposal (perhaps for a PhD fellowship application; see below).

PhD training

PhD scholarships

PhD scholarships are normally for three years full time. Universities may be offered a number of government-funded PhD scholarships (which include a tax free amount for subsistence (£12,000) plus fees and an annual stipend for training, approximately £1,000) for which physiotherapists can apply. Normally awards are very competitive, and will be awarded to the students with the best degree qualifications. Masters level qualifications can improve an applicants chances of being awarded a PhD scholarship, especially if they are in a similar field of study. Some universities may have separate awards on offer, for example: the university-funded Vice Chancellor Scholarship Scheme at the University of Ulster or studentships resulting from the awards of external grant funding to the university from charities, industry and so on.

PhD fellowship schemes

If you are employed in the health service, the relevant NHS Research and Development (R&D) office may provide funding for you to complete a PhD, at a suitable collaborating academic institution, for either three years on a full-time basis or five years on a part-time basis. The fellowship normally pays your health service salary, your PhD fees and training expenses. These fellowships are very competitive and require submission of a full research proposal for the PhD (in Northern Ireland, **http://www.centralservicesagency.com/display/rdo_education_training2**).

For some schemes you will need to ensure that you have already made a link with at least one academic supervisor who is willing to supervise your PhD. This person can also help guide you in writing your research proposal and thus increase your chances of getting the fellowship. A recent initiative in Northern Ireland by the R&D office has been the establishment of learning sets which aim to provide expert academic guidance, to nursing and therapy clinicians, on the completion of their research proposal and fellowship form.

Information on PhD-funded vacancies can be accessed via the following website: **http://www.jobs.ac.uk/jobtype/student/** Some of these PhDs will be in departments or groups led by physiotherapists; others may not, but the topic area may be very relevant to physiotherapy practice, so they are worth exploring.

You could also obtain information from your local university. Normally, funded scholarships are advertised at the beginning of the year for a September/October start. However if you can self-fund, it may be possible to apply for PhD training at any time of the year. Note that practice varies from one university to another.

Making the right networks

It is very important to remember that the strongest clinical research is always done in teams; it is unlikely that it is even possible for an individual to carry out high quality clinical research alone. So you need to think about how you can make networks with colleagues both inside your own department, and elsewhere in your clinical setting.

Consider the following:
- Think about local academic centres that can provide expert research guidance, and which may already be carrying out research in your area of interest.

- Try to establish what research is being carried out in your own department. Do you have a joint appointment with the local university? If so, this person should be able to guide you to appropriate academic contacts. Are there people in your department who are carrying out a research project? Speak to them and find out how they did it: it may be that they are on a PhD fellowship (see PhD training above) or completing a masters.

- Another good starting point would be your hospital R&D office which should be able to help you identify people to network with on site.

- Try your NHS R&D office which can let you know if there are already established networks in your area. For example in Northern Ireland, the NI R&D office supports a number of Recognised Research Groups (RRGs), one of which is the Trauma and Rehabilitation RRG. Membership of this RRG is open to all and contains academics and clinicians from a wide range of disciplines, including physiotherapists. Information about this RRG can be found at **http://www.centralservicesagency. com/display/rdo_research_groups**. It provides an excellent forum for a novice researcher to get involved with more established clinical researchers, who are usually more than willing to provide mentorship.

- Other ways of making networks are to join a research society (such as the Physiotherapy Research Society (PRS), or to become part a support network such as the National Physiotherapy Research Network (NPRN).

Pump priming funding

Success in achieving research funding depends upon an established track record in funding. So how do you get funding if you have no track record and no real research experience? Again the key is to network with an experienced research team, and make sure you are aware of funding specifically targeted at novice researchers. There are many organisations which specifically aim to provide small amounts of funding for novice researchers who are working within an experienced team of researchers.

This funding is sometimes called 'seed' or 'pump prime' funding as the idea is to enable a novice researcher to complete some exploratory work that could then be used as the basis of a further, larger grant application. In physiotherapy the CSP's PRF takes on this role. The PRF provides ring-fenced funding for novice members of the CSP to carry out their first piece of funded research. Other sources of pump priming can be found at RD info **(http://www.rdinfo.org.uk/)**; it helps to search this site under your clinical area of interest. Many charitable organisations, clinical support groups or CSP special interest groups will be able to fund small projects (£1,000–£5,000) to get you going!

Prioritise research

Unless you are extremely disciplined about identifying time to do research as part of your clinical post, it is very unlikely that you will be successful. There are several ways that you can improve your chances of being successful in setting aside some time for research:
- Get a small grant to cover some of your clinical time so that you can dedicate this time to your research (see pump prime funding).
- Discuss with your line manager any strategies that the department has in place to support clinical research. Discuss the possibilities of setting up joint appointments with the local university to support clinical research.
- Apply to do a masters programme, as this will give you a structured target to work towards and will help you prioritise your time. You may be able to negotiate some time off from your manager to support attendance at a masters programme.
- Apply for a fellowship to complete your MPhil or PhD on a full-time or part-time basis.
- Apply for funds to complete a professional doctorate: these are usually part-time programmes.

Reference list
- Research Training in the Healthcare Professions. Report produced by the UK Council for Graduate Education (2003). **http://www.ukcge.ac.uk/NR/rdonlyres/ F3EFB9F9-3FD0-45A4-869A-2B0A97B0D858/0/HealthcareProfessions200 3.pdf**

- Strategic Learning and Research (StLaR) HR Plan Project. Supporting learning and research in health and social care. **http://www.stlarhr.org.uk**

2.3 Registering on a professional doctorate programme
Nikki Petty

What is a professional doctorate? ~ the programme ~ managing your time ~ assessment ~ financing your studies ~ a personal experience

What is a professional doctorate?

It is a doctoral research degree, equivalent to a PhD, which aims to develop researching professionals. Doctoral programmes around the country vary in their format and structure.

How is the programme delivered?
Programmes are usually delivered part-time with yearly cohorts of students. The programme normally lasts between four to six years.

Will the programme be just for physiotherapists?
Student cohorts are usually from a variety of health professions such as nursing, midwifery, occupational therapy, podiatry, and physiotherapy. In addition, students may be working in a variety of practice settings, including clinical, management and higher education.

How is the programme structured?
Programmes are usually structured around regular study days and this provides the educational arm to the professional doctorate. Later on in the programme the student starts the research arm to the doctorate, with the allocation of a research supervisor and regular supervisory meetings.

What happens on study days?
The student cohort meets regularly together for study days lasting one or two days. During this time there may be teaching and discussion sessions on particular aspects underpinning research, such as methodology, methods, ethics and data analysis, as well as action learning sets and tutorial support. It may also include computer and library support sessions to support electronic literature searches, referencing software, data analysis software and guidance on creating long documents.

What happens between study days?
You need to study on your own!

How do I manage my time?
Being organised with your time and making the doctorate a priority is probably one of the most important things you need to do. Careful consideration of how you can maintain a healthy work-life balance is needed to sustain the level of effort required over the prolonged period of time.

You probably need to find about one day a week to study consistently over the four-year period; towards the end of the programme when you're writing up the thesis you may need to find extended periods of time. If you are employed you may need to negotiate time from your employer and it is worth being well prepared for this discussion. As you progress through the programme you may need to renegotiate your time. Being flexible, assertive and resilient will all facilitate this process.

How is the doctorate assessed?
There are usually written assignments given at particular stages of the programme and students may be supported by an advisor. As an example one programme has four assignments. The first is identifying a researchable problem (6,000 words); second is exploring appropriate methodologies (8,000 words); third is a small scale pilot study (12,000 words) and the fourth is the final thesis of a research study involving professional practice (50,000 words) followed by a viva. The student receives doctoral credits after successful completion of each assignment and this finally adds up to the doctoral award with 540 credits. This staged feedback helps to develop the students' competence and confidence as researchers as they move towards the final hurdle of the thesis and viva.

What will the professional doctorate do for me?
Doctoral programmes will enable you to become a competent researcher in your professional practice and therefore enhance your skills in generating research knowledge relevant to practice and in using evidence-informed practice. To achieve this, the programme will provide an educational package that will develop your research knowledge and skills and with the support of supervisors, you will then research an aspect of your professional practice.

Am I eligible to apply?
Normally, if you are a chartered physiotherapist with HPC registration, have gained a few years of professional experience, and have a masters-level degree then you are able to apply. You don't normally have to know your research topic before coming onto the course, but being able to discuss your ideas will be necessary at interview.

2.3

What are the financial costs?
There are a variety of costs involved including:
- annual cost for the programme.
- travel and accommodation costs to attend the study days and supervisory meetings.
- purchasing books and articles.
- reprographics.
- costs related to carrying out the research, for example digital recorders.
- professional proofreader.
- printing and binding the thesis.

Are there any grants available to me to do a professional doctorate?
The Chartered Society of Physiotherapy (CSP) offers educational grants, as do clinical interest groups such as the Manipulation Association of Chartered Society of Physiotherapists (MACP). Contact the organisation to gain up-to-date information and guidance on applying for a grant.

Where are professional doctorate programmes run for physiotherapists?
The first named professional doctorate in physiotherapy in the UK was set up in 2003 in the School of Health Professions, University of Brighton. Since then a number of courses have sprung up around the country. A Google search or a search of the CSP website will readily identify the current courses available.

A personal experience of completing a professional doctorate in physiotherapy

I can summarise the whole experience by saying it was a fantastic mid-life refreshment. I had been enjoying my work in higher education for 12 years, teaching undergraduate and postgraduate students. I had become fascinated by postgraduate teaching and the way students changed during the MSc neuromusculoskeletal physiotherapy course at the University of Brighton. Having spent years reflecting on my own teaching practice, I wanted to explore and research the process from the students' point of view. My career and professional aspirations were centred on the process of learning and teaching, this was what I really enjoyed doing at work. As I knew that a professional doctorate would help me research my practice within higher education, it was more attractive to me than a PhD. I was also attracted to the structure and format, with progressive assignments that provided clear feedback on my development. The peer cohort group of health professionals provided a broader perspective, an opportunity for friendships, and much needed emotional support!

Looking back at the course now, I can honestly say the structure and format did what I expected it to do. The progressive assignments gave focus to studying and a gradual step-by-step sense of development. One unexpected surprise was that once I handed in an assignment, I completely switched off from my studying until I received my mark; it was as if all my motivation and drive had been put on hold. This provided some respite and also enabled me to do some rather major DIY projects around the house, including redecoration of my study! Getting the pass mark and thorough feedback on an assignment then boosted my confidence; it also gave plenty of food for thought that got me back into studying. After the third assignment, there was a subtle difference as I realised the final assignment was now the big THESIS!

I'm writing this chapter while still completing the professional doctorate programme. I am at the moment writing chapters of the thesis and hope to complete within a total of five academic years. I can't tell you yet how the final part of writing goes or what the viva was like; those are stories for another time. But for now I can honestly say it has been the best learning experience I have ever had. I would wholeheartedly recommend this sort of programme to you.

2.4 Registering on a traditional PhD programme
Liz Cousins

What is a traditional PhD? ~ the programme ~ supervision ~ funding ~ ethics ~ the key stages ~ how it can contribute to career development ~ a personal view

What is a traditional PhD?
A traditional PhD is a higher degree achieved through the completion of an original piece of research, the writing up of this research as a thesis, and finally an oral defence of your work with other academics. A PhD is effectively a qualification in research, which shows that the individual who has successfully completed a PhD is capable of carrying out independent research.

How is the programme delivered?
PhDs can be completed on either a full or part-time basis. Typically, a full-time PhD is expected to last for three years, while part-time PhDs are normally expected to be completed in up to six years.

What is the role of a supervisor?
When you register on a traditional PhD programme, you will be allocated a supervisor, or a team of supervisors. Their role is to oversee your programme of research, guide you through the processes involved, working to keep your PhD on track. They are there to ensure that your research, critical thinking and written work are of the standard required for doctoral study. In addition to academic work, they may help with administrative issues and personal support. They are not however there to do the PhD for you, and the onus is on the individual registered for the PhD to take the steps that are required for the successful completion of the thesis.

What qualifications are required?
The minimum requirement is usually a 1st or 2:1 in an undergraduate degree. A masters degree is not essential, although it may well be advantageous in an application for a PhD, as it provides evidence of academic work at a higher level.

How do I start on a traditional PhD?
Funded PhDs are occasionally advertised locally or through the relevant professional press. However, if you are interested in doing a self-funded PhD your first port of call should be a university department. Although you may well have some ideas of what you might want to research as your PhD, early discussions with a potential supervisor

will help ascertain the feasibility of your plans. Even if you don't have any specific ideas for research that you want to incorporate into a PhD, lecturers in the university know where their expertise lies and what facilities are available at the university. Discussion with them may well lead into the development of a project that could form the basis of a PhD.

Funding for PhD

Funding for a PhD may come from internal sources at the university, or as part of a successful bid for a research grant from an external source. Funding for a full-time PhD is typically for a three-year period. Even if there is no available funding for a PhD when you first contact a potential supervisor, it may be that support for a research degree could be included as part of a future funding bid. This is another reason why, if you're considering undertaking a PhD, it is worth contacting potential supervisors (or departments) as a first step, rather than waiting for a PhD programme to be advertised. Alternatively, students can self-fund.

Ethics

All research involving people will need some sort of ethical approval. As physiotherapists, the original piece of research for your PhD may well involve patients within the NHS, and this will require ethical approval from NRES. The processes of gaining ethical approval are discussed in another chapter of this book, but it is worth noting that the time taken to get through these processes should not be underestimated. It is not unheard of for these procedures to take more than a year to complete: a substantial length of time if you only have funding for three years of study. However the systems are becoming more streamlined and your supervisors will be able to advise you throughout the process.

2.4

What can I expect during a traditional PhD programme?

A typical PhD programme can be subdivided into several parts, as follows:
- formal research training.
- background reading.
- formulation of a research proposal and designing the study.
- gaining necessary ethical approvals.

The first part of a traditional PhD is incredibly important. Errors made at this stage (for example in the design of your study) cannot always be rectified later. It is very important to gain thorough background knowledge of the literature and to explore facilities available to you at the university and how these can be incorporated into your research. For example, what equipment is available for you to use during your data collection? Alternatively, what equipment or resources may need to be acquired, or what software packages are around that you may want to use in the subsequent analysis of this data? It is therefore possible that even if you begin your PhD study with a clear idea of the research you want to undertake, it may be some time before you actually begin the research studies themselves.

Data collection and analysis
Once the preliminary work is completed, the actual research study (or studies) can be undertaken.

Writing up
This is the translation of the entire research project into one cohesive document that can subsequently be examined.

Examination
A PhD is awarded after the successful completion of a written thesis and a viva voce (oral) examination, by at least two chosen examiners. There is always at least one examiner who is external to the university at which you're registered, and sometimes all the examiners will be external. Essentially, the examiners will discuss the thesis with you in depth. There is no single standard format for a viva, but the examiners will seek to ask you questions about the research, your chosen methodologies, and to explore your conclusions. Above all they will need to confirm that the work submitted is indeed your work, and that the appropriate level has been achieved. Following the viva the examiners may recommend you for the awarding of a PhD outright, or following minor changes to the thesis. They can also ask for major revisions of the

thesis to be completed before they will recommend that it be passed. It is also possible to be awarded an MPhil instead of a PhD under certain circumstances, or to be failed outright.

Are there any other formal processes I need to go through as part of a traditional PhD?

There are a number of formal processes you need to go through as part of a traditional PhD, which have to be completed before you can even submit your thesis. A PhD is a higher degree with a specific aim of research training. As such, it is expected that students registered for a PhD will also undergo courses, during their programme of study, that will contribute to their research training. In some universities it is compulsory to complete a certain number of credits in taught modules that contribute to the student's research training (for example research methods or statistics). If you have already completed a masters degree, or stand alone M-level modules, this may contribute to your research training, and you may find you don't need to get as many credits as a PhD student who only has an undergraduate degree. The opportunity to undertake specific courses in areas relevant to your research is an excellent one, and even if your specific university does not require completion of such modules, it is highly recommended. Usually, the majority of the formal research training that you undertake would be completed within the first year of doctoral study. In addition to the above formal research training that you may have to undertake, there is often a transfer process that students have to go through, this being the official conversion of the student's registration status from that of MPhil/PhD, to that of PhD. In order to achieve this transfer of status, the student has to demonstrate that they are suitable for, and capable of successfully completing a doctoral study, and that the thesis will achieve doctoral level. The exact process students have to go through will vary depending on the university at which they are registered, but will normally include a piece of written work based on the research done to date, and a viva. The transfer process usually takes place at the end of the first year of full-time study, and is taken very seriously by universities who consider it an important part of the PhD.

How can a traditional PhD contribute to career development?

A PhD is obviously a valuable (and sometimes essential) qualification to have if you want to pursue a career in academia or research. A PhD can also make a considerable contribution to a clinical career. The PhD leads to greater understanding of a specific area, but there are many skills broader than this which would have a direct influence

2.4

on clinical work, for example the ability to analyse and understand the clinical processes you go through, the questioning that becomes second nature as part of a PhD, and the ability to appraise literature and apply it to clinical situations. In a world demanding evidence-based practice, these skills are invaluable. Additionally, successful completion of a PhD demonstrates the ability to work independently and the organisational skills that are essential to all areas of work.

Personal view

Prior to my PhD I was working as a lead practitioner in neurology and rehabilitation in a district general hospital. My motivation in going into research was to understand more fully the clinical work I was doing, and the changes that I saw in the patients we treated. The PhD I am currently undertaking had received internal funding from the university, and was advertised in the national physiotherapy press. It was in an area that I was particularly interested in, so I approached the supervisor for more information. I didn't have a masters degree, and any research experience was limited to my undergraduate degree, so I have to admit to being shocked to be offered the studentship! It does go to show however, that all applications will be considered by a university. The journey through this PhD has certainly been challenging, yet it is also the most rewarding and exciting work I have done to date. Low points for me were getting the ethical approval necessary to begin one of my research studies: it took me more than a year just to be allowed to start! A direct consequence of this was an enforced delay to my studies. Highlights would have to be data collecting and working with the participants on the studies. Their interest and enthusiasm for the research never ceased to amaze me, and their dedication to the various projects was astounding. At the present time, my data collection has been completed, and I am now in the process of analysing the work and writing the thesis. While I do not yet know where this PhD will lead me career-wise, I am confident that the research skills I have learnt over the past few years will be useful, and that I will be able to fully integrate them into whichever job I end up in.

Life after completing a PhD   2.5
Brona McDowell

As a physiotherapist on rotation ~ in a joint research appointment ~ as a clinical researcher ~ a personal perspective - rewards and challenges

Completing my PhD

Completing a PhD can open up many new avenues regarding career direction, many of which are discussed within the chapters of this book. I enrolled on a full-time PhD studentship directly after completing my undergraduate degree and on completion of my thesis, worked as a physiotherapist within the NHS. I then spent three years in a joint research appointment and for the last seven years have worked as a clinical researcher, primarily in the area of paediatric orthopaedics. In this chapter I have been asked to share my experience of life after completing a PhD. Many others will have had a very different experience.

As a physiotherapist on rotation

Job-hunting in the NHS isn't necessarily any easier with a PhD, especially if one has gone straight into a research programme as a new graduate. A doctorate counts for little when competing against new graduates well versed in interview techniques and in this respect, being out of the loop for three years isn't an advantage! Alternatively, whilst completing a PhD, maintaining ones clinical skills by undertaking part-time work in the evenings and at weekends, is to be recommended. It allows one to maintain, practise and become more proficient in the clinical skills gained during training and keep abreast of any changes in practice. It is also an advantage when looking for more senior posts further down the line.

In a joint research appointment

Joint research appointments are one form of clinical academic posts formed as a partnership between an NHS trust and a university. These posts allow for clinical time within a specialist clinical service and research time, often on a designated research project. A limited amount of teaching is often included within the job description. There are many positive aspects to these types of posts. The intrinsic link with a university provides much of the academic support that is necessary for getting a research project started; writing grants, gaining ethical approval and so on, while the link with the trust makes it easier to liaise with relevant clinical staff, obtain research sponsorship and access patients for recruitment. Working on a university site also affords one the camaraderie of other colleagues working in similar areas of rehabilitation research.

On the negative side, the roles and responsibilities within these posts are often vast, and having designated time for each is often unrealistic, particularly as the post evolves. If teaching duties are written into the contract this also takes away from the time that can be dedicated to research, particularly within the first year. Being responsible to two line managers, with regard to job performance and staff appraisal, can also at times be challenging, particularly if research priorities differ. University-held contracts are more commonly fixed term and thus job security may be an additional concern. Regardless, these types of posts offer an excellent way of getting a foothold in research while, at the same time, maintaining ones clinical skills. They also provide a useful stepping-stone for anyone interested in pursuing a more permanent academic career.

As a clinical researcher

These types of posts can take many forms and my own experience comes from working as a clinical specialist with some dedicated time for research activity. On a weekly, and often daily basis, time is juggled between clinical and research responsibilities, and the time dedicated to each will often depend on the specific post. Vying for large research grants relies on having a substantial research portfolio, thus the early years may often be spent carrying out small pilot and feasibility studies. For many, this will involve collecting the data oneself, although local research awards/bursaries and smaller grants may enable the recruitment of another clinician/researcher to assist. Compared with posts linked to academic institutions, life as a clinical researcher can be a more isolated one, especially if there are no other clinical researchers within the department and limited research structures within the trust. There are number of ways of easing this and getting your research kick-started:

- Maintain any existing links with academic partners and work at establishing new ones. Such links are vital when competing for large external sources of funding and supervising potential research students.
- Join a local recognised research group or network that has research themes relevant to your area. These groups can provide much needed support and access to small amounts of funding.
- Avail yourself of any support networks in your area. Many NHS regions now have established clinical research and trials units: these units often provide clinical researchers with one-to-one advice on designing a project, working out a statistical plan, writing a grant proposal and gaining ethical approval. They also run courses that may be of benefit.

- Make links with other clinical research centres that may potentially act as collaborators on future research projects. If working as a sole clinical specialist in a geographical region, such links are important and are best achieved by attending conferences of mutual interest.

Ever-increasing bureaucracy has made life as a clinical researcher more demanding and more rigorous guidelines contained within the Research Governance Framework, pertaining to Good Clinical Practice, ethical approval and research sponsorship, has made research a less attractive option for many clinicians. Despite this, it still represents an interesting career option for anyone who really loves working as a clinician but also has an interest in conducting research.

A personal perspective – rewards and challenges

A career in research offers many challenges, not least because the goals keep changing. For example, within the field of rehabilitation medicine, concepts such as participation and quality of life present a whole new challenge in terms of assessing outcome. For many, including myself, this forms much of the appeal. Many days spent in research are frustrating; sorting out administration, wading through data or writing a paper that just doesn't seem to be going anywhere, while other days are rewarding; receiving ethical approval, getting a paper accepted for publication or positive feedback from patients and their families. By far, one of the most rewarding aspects of the job has been supervising students, and I have now supervised several colleagues through to completion of MPhil and PhD study through close links with local Universities. Juggling a career in research with having a family has definitely been one of my greatest challenges, not least because I work part-time. In order to maintain an adequate research portfolio, many tasks, such as reviewing papers, grants and theses, often have to be taken home: attending conferences and meetings also means time spent away from the family.

Carrying out a PhD has allowed me to follow an altogether different career path than any I would have envisioned as an undergraduate and, even though my thesis was not in an area of personal interest, I thoroughly valued the research training it provided. I used my years working as a junior physiotherapist to identify a clinical area of interest and, for the last ten years, have undertaken a clinical role within the field of gait analysis and a research role, primarily in the area of paediatric orthopaedics. Working in a joint research appointment

2.5

was an excellent way of getting involved in clinical research, while, working within the NHS has afforded me greater job security and the flexibility to work part-time. Within the health service I have also had the added benefit of line management that has promoted research within the department and offered good impartial advice and support when needed; this has been an invaluable resource over the years. I continue to enjoy my clinical remit, which mainly involves the assessment of children with disabilities, and hope that the research contribution I make in this field over the years will in some way contribute to a better knowledge base, improved rehabilitation methods and a better lifestyle in this population of young people.

The route from novice to Principal Investigator

2.6

Di Newham

What is a Principal Investigator (PI)? ~ what is a PI responsible for? ~ what is a novice researcher? ~ what are the possible routes from novice researcher to PI ~ PhD ~ postdoctoral work?

What is a Principal Investigator?

The term Principal Investigator (PI) refers to a senior researcher who takes the lead role in a particular research project and they are always identified on a grant application to fund research. They will have been instrumental in developing the original idea, bringing the collaborators together, developing the protocol and writing grant applications.

PIs are usually regarded as leading experts in their field and at least will be well known in their field as a result of their research publications, presentations at meeting and perhaps authorship of books or chapters in books. They have built up over a number of years a curriculum vitae (CV) that shows a considerable number of research publications in the form of original research papers in well respected journals and abstracts from presentations at meetings and also having been awarded research funding either as the PI or a named applicant.

What is a PI responsible for?

A PI often has a number of research projects active at any one time, are most if not all of these will have funding. They will be leading a team of people involving PhD students and postdoctoral workers. As a result of their previous work they will have built up a number of collaborators. They will be constantly seeking new collaborators as research ideas develop and change, often demanding the expertise of people from other disciplines.

When a project is running the PI has overall responsibility for it. This covers every aspect of the project from subject recruitment to the preparation of publications. If a project funds research staff or students the PI is also responsible for them and will usually be their line manager. If a PhD student is involved in the project the PI will normally be one of their supervisors.

All but the smallest research projects require funding and all grant applications require a named PI. Usually there are a number of other named applicants who are colleagues of the applicant and who have a clearly defined role, and perhaps different types of expertise in the research itself. They will also have been involved developing the research question, design and preparation of the application.

Some people working in a clinical setting may well have years of research experience that involved working on projects for which they were neither the PI nor a named applicant. Some of these could be undertaken without any specific research funding. The driver in this situation is the interest in the research itself and usually publishing the findings, but the role of PI may not be viewed as an important goal or achievement. The situation in universities is different as academic staff are expected to achieve PI status in order to be able to attract research funding and build up their teams of PhD students, research assistants and postdoctoral researchers.

What is a novice researcher?

A novice researcher is someone who wishes to be involved in research but who has little or no research knowledge, experience or skills. Clinicians who have qualified with university degrees will usually have undertaken a research project which will give some insight and direct experience of research but cannot equip anyone to the stage of being able to be an independent researcher, let alone a PI. Novice researchers and PIs are essentially at opposite ends of the spectrum of research expertise. There are many steps from one to the other and naturally not all researchers will choose to move to the PI end of the spectrum.

What are the possible routes from novice researcher to PI?

The purpose of this chapter is to provide some information about ways to move from the position of a novice researcher towards that of a PI. There is no single route for this, although there is a traditional one for people in academic university departments. The key for progression is the acquisition of research skills and knowledge that enable an individual to have good, original research ideas that they can work up into questions and protocols that will generate data worthy of publication and able to attract research funding. This will inevitably involve collaboration with others, often from different disciplines or with specific skills or knowledge.

2.6

The traditional, formal academic route towards becoming a PI is hierarchical and involves the achievement of a good classification undergraduate degree followed by postgraduate study at the level of masters then PhD work and finally postdoctoral experience. In this model the PhD and postdoctoral work is done on a full-time basis and supported by research grants obtained by the PhD supervisor. Those at postdoctoral level will start to be involved in submitting research grants which could involve being a named researcher whose salary will be paid by the grant as well as being a named applicant.

This route is not necessarily followed by allied health professionals who wish to develop their research career, perhaps to the level of PI. Many graduates wish to gain some clinical experience before pursuing their research activities. During this time they may well become involved in local research projects, gaining valuable experience and perhaps becoming an author on the resulting publications. They may wish to follow CPD activities that are research related and may involve studying at masters level on individual modules or for a masters degree, either full or part-time. Professional doctorates are a more recent way of gaining relevant experience and knowledge.

Which ever route is followed, the constant and key issue is the need for mentors who are already at the PI stage or close to it. Formal mentoring is undertaken by the supervisors of masters and doctoral work although informal mentoring and support by people with more experience is essential for all researchers. This includes experienced PIs who are usually very aware of the importance of input from those with greater experience.

PhD

Normally a PI will have been awarded a PhD some years previously and in the intervening time will have continued to develop their research career by being involved in grant applications and publishing their research findings. This provides the opportunity to develop the skills and expertise to become an independent researcher. These can be developed more informally over a number of years of research experience, but the formal supervision and requirements for the award of a PhD provide a nationally recognised standard of research knowledge and experience as well as a commitment to developing a research career, whether this is in a clinical or academic setting.
In well established subjects in universities a PhD is the minimum qualification for an

academic post in a university. In the newly emerging academic disciplines, such as the allied health professions there still relatively few people with a PhD, although the number of people with this qualification is steadily rising in physiotherapy. This is a healthy sign of the academic development of the profession.

When physiotherapy first became a graduate entry profession, there were not enough physiotherapists with a PhD to fill the academic posts in university departments of physiotherapy. In the more research oriented institutions staff were frequently appointed on the basis of their academic/research potential and were expected to obtain a PhD as part of their employment conditions. As the number of physiotherapists with a PhD increases, this qualification is being increasingly seen as a basic requirement for a university position.

For those who wish to develop their research career in a clinical setting a PhD still has some advantages. One reason is that it is an academic currency indicating an agreed level of intellectual ability along with an accepted level of research skills and experience. The people from other disciplines that they are working with will most likely have a PhD and, rightly or wrongly, may think that someone who does not is less skilled and working at a lower level.

PhD studies involve the equivalent of three years' full-time research or six years' part-time, writing a thesis and an oral examination with at least two examiners (see chapters 2.4 and 2.5). They are an early step on the path from novice researcher to PI. While some publications usually result from the research undertaken, the individual will have worked under close supervision at all stages of the programme.

The award of a PhD does not mean that people have the necessary skills and experience to immediately become a PI. To be able to undertake this role normally takes a further few years of active research and the establishment of a reputation in the particular field.

Postdoctoral work

Having acquired basic research training as part of their PhD studies, a career researcher needs to consolidate their knowledge and experience. This still involves working with one or more PIs whose experience is necessary in a mentoring role and who are in a position to be able to attract research funding so that the research can continue.

2.6

The postdoctoral researcher has more autonomy than a PhD student and indeed they are often involved in working with and supporting such students and less experienced researchers. Formal supervision of PhD students is not normally undertaken until someone has several years of postdoctoral research experience. Even then they should only take on a secondary supervisory role while the primary one is taken by someone with previous experience of PhD supervision.

This can be done in the more formal and traditional way by working full-time in the position of postdoctoral researcher. This invariably involves working on a project for which funding has been acquired by someone well established as a PI and in this case the project will have been fully worked up for the grant application.

Alternatively the postdoctoral worker may have been involved in the formulation of the research question and development of the project and also perhaps writing funding applications.

Essentially the two options are to continue working with the same group of people involved in the PhD work or to join another group. There is no fixed position on which route is best. However working with another group of people does offer the opportunity for experience of different research approaches and methodologies along with the possibility of learning new techniques.

2.7 A senior physiotherapist with a postgraduate masters degree: developing research interests
Janet Deane

What is a postgraduate masters degree ~ course structure ~ why begin an MSc ~ developing research interests ~ the research question ~ the research proposal ~ how can I develop research interests beyond the MSc ~ researcher skills ~ can I combine research and clinical work?

What is a postgraduate masters degree?

A postgraduate masters degree or MSc is designed to enable physiotherapists and other allied professionals to develop their full professional, educational and research potential within their clinical field.

The postgraduate masters degree develops an advanced knowledge of the research base that underpins current practice, and refines existing practical skills through clinical placement and supervised practical sessions with expert clinicians. It also develops existing analytical and reflective skills, which enable one to formulate and carry out an independent research study with confidence.

All of these skills, in the current climate of evidence-based practice and professional accountability, help ensure the highest standard of healthcare and professional satisfaction.

The entry requirements vary from university to university but it is usually best to have approximately four to five years of clinical experience before applying, in order to gain the maximum benefit. This is largely because MSc programmes assume a certain baseline level of knowledge and clinical experience, which is then used as a platform to develop expertise or masters level knowledge in a given area.

What is the usual course structure?
An MSc is usually structured around several distinct modules but this may vary depending on the university. In my experience, the programme consisted of both obligatory and optional modules, comprising of a mixture of theoretical and practical units, which meant that there was plenty of opportunity to indulge and explore areas of personal interest.

Why begin an MSc?
As a physiotherapist with a background in science, I wished to engage these two aspects of my past and present. Working as a clinician in physiotherapy, as in other allied health

professions, one finds oneself continually asking questions for which there are not always answers.

Increasingly, during rotations as a junior and senior physiotherapist, I found myself asking questions and trying to establish possible answers. Although I found continuing professional development sessions, teaching and engaging in various mini-research projects interesting, there came a point in my career where I felt a further academic challenge was necessary, in order to gain specialist knowledge, develop advanced research skills and progress in my career.

By completing an MSc in advanced musculoskeletal physiotherapy, I was able to explore personal research interests freely while developing my full potential within the field of musculoskeletal physiotherapy.

Developing research interests

Research interests can develop from the smallest idea or thought. Most allied health professionals find that their best ideas are conceived while treating patients, attending lectures or simply through reading or discussing research with colleagues.

As a junior practitioner or novice, it is common to be hesitant in expressing ideas or questions because one feels that the knowledge of respected colleagues is far greater. However, be assured that all questions and ideas are valuable and it is only through asking these questions that the profession evolves, research interests develop and healthcare improves.

How do I develop an idea into a research question?

Firstly, in my experience, the main problems people encounter when first developing an idea is the failure to develop a simple, achievable research question. One can collect endless data in haste to proceed with a project, but without a concise, specific and achievable objective, the data collected may be largely useless.

Secondly, I have found it very important to develop a research question in an area in which you have a real interest. Although, this seems intuitive, it is this interest that you will find carries you through the ups and downs of your research study and motivates and drives you forwards even when you feel like giving up.
On the MSc programme I undertook at University College London, I was encouraged to

2.7

develop a research question shortly after beginning the course. I found that by establishing a concise question early on, it narrowed the subsequent literature review I had to carry out. This in turn meant I could develop a succinct research proposal ready for peer and ethical review in good time, so that I was capable of committing myself fully to the other modules required by my programme.

Before you can proceed with your study, a peer review or evaluation of your proposal is required by an expert in the field, in order to determine whether the study is relevant and realistic. It is also vital to go through the necessary ethical approval processes. Depending on the nature of your study, applications for ethical approval might be considered by a university committee, or by an NHS research ethics committees. Approval can take up to six months to obtain, emphasising again the necessity of organisation and forward planning.

What happens after a research proposal has been approved?

After your proposal has been given approval the wheels are then set in motion for you to begin your study. Again, being realistic with the initial protocol is important, especially on a full-time MSc programme.

On a full time programme you have approximately six months from the conception of the idea to research completion and write up. This means that commitment and determination are required in large quantities. I found that in order to keep on top of it all, it was important to consistently chip away at it rather than leaving it all to the last minute, which may lead to a lot of unnecessary panic close to the final examinations.

How can I develop research interests beyond the MSc?

Since qualifying, I have become a member of various clinical interest groups and have regular contact with physiotherapists who have similar clinical interests. This can really help to foster new ideas and provides a supportive environment in which you can progress as a researcher. Through the MSc programme it is possible to develop a diverse network of clinical contacts, which becomes extremely useful in the world of research. It is largely through these people that you become aware of job opportunities, ideas for career progression and may even be approached to assist with other projects.

Since completing my MSc I have taken on a research physiotherapist post at Imperial College, which means that I now work with a team of researchers on a large clinical study. In this position I am surrounded by healthcare professionals from different backgrounds who are taking part in a range of projects: this means I continue to learn as a researcher almost by osmosis!

What skills do I require to become a researcher?

In my experience, a researcher requires an inquisitive and methodical nature, a supportive environment, courage and a lot of persistence!

A deep interest in the subject matter being researched also helps. As I have mentioned before, it is this interest that drives you to completion, particularly with larger studies.

I strongly believe that we, as physiotherapists, are continuously researching and therefore have a lot of the required skills. The only difficulty is that because we do it on a daily basis we do not always credit our ideas or small projects as research. As a result our innovation goes unnoticed as we do not feel equipped to voice our findings and take it to the next level. The MSc, in my opinion, helps to grow the confidence required to develop a research idea or interest into a research study: one that might be presented and published. The experience of this process certainly forms a solid base from which a career in research can be built.

Can I combine research and clinical work?

It is possible to work as a full or part-time researcher in the allied health professions. At present, I combine my work as a research physiotherapist with that of a private musculoskeletal practitioner. I find this has achieved the right balance for me as I am able to apply evolving research findings to my current clinical work and at the same time use my work as a clinician to generate new research ideas.

In time to come I might seek further challenges in the form of a PhD, and even become a full-time researcher, but for now I feel quite content to enjoy the diversity that my current career as a physiotherapist offers me.

2.8 Contract research staff roles
Sally Singh

Junior contract researcher ~ senior contract researcher ~ professor of physiotherapy ~ lecturer ~ clinical researcher ~ research consultant ~ the research-orientated manager

This chapter will define the roles and responsibilities of various contract research roles. Traditionally these have been accommodated within universities, but there are emerging roles as either joint appointments with NHS organisations or for research to be hosted by the healthcare provider with supervision from within that organisation. Frequently these posts are offered as a fixed-term contract.

Each role will be explored separately but there will be common themes to allow comparison and progression through the research hierarchy. These will include the required experience for the posts, supervisory skills and leadership qualities.

Junior contract researcher

These posts are usually associated with a specific project for which there is funding and the details of the project formulated. The post will be supervised by a senior researcher. The post will usually require the holder to have a good honours degree (at least a 2:1) or a relevant professional qualification. It is advantageous to have some clinical experience/knowledge of the subject area. Frequently these posts involve routine data collection and data entry. These tasks carry considerable responsibility and work is frequently completed independently. Good keyboard and limited data interpretation skills would be required with a working knowledge of computerised statistical analysis programmes. The post holder should have the necessary writing skills to compose abstracts and be developing presentation skills.

Senior contract researcher

Senior researchers are required to have a good degree and relevant professional experience in the area of the project. The researcher at this level would be expected to demonstrate a detailed knowledge of the subject area being investigated and have some research experience. This experience would be beyond that acquired at undergraduate level and possibly acquired formally as a junior contract researcher or clinical researcher. The researcher at this level should be able to write protocols and operationalise them, including overseeing the ethics procedure. The post would require the holder to establish and guarantee quality assurance procedures and ensure the integrity of the data in accordance with data protection legislation. Consequently the senior researcher should be able to generate data and conduct the appropriate analysis of a sufficient standard to generate abstracts for presentation at local, national or international conferences. This would necessitate good analytical and writing skills. This person should have the skills to write research reports and prepare manuscripts. In addition the role would require input to the development of new research ideas and the preparation of research proposals. The post is supervised but should allow the post holder to develop their own supervisory and leadership skills. The senior researcher should also be developing research networks within the UK and beyond.

Professor of Physiotherapy

A Professor of Physiotherapy has overall responsibility for a programme of research. Inevitably the role requires the post holder to hold a PhD and have significant clinical and research experience in the specified area of research. This should be supported by an extensive publication record, of original research in peer-reviewed journals. This is supported by other research outputs including editorials, reviews and book chapters. This post requires demonstrable presentation skills with experience at national and international conferences and thus the post holder should carry a national/international reputation. In addition to presenting at significant meetings a Professor should be required to chair sessions of scientific presentations and facilitate productive and concise discussions. The professor attracts important research project funding. The role also requires the ability to manage a team of research staff. The post holder should also be a strong team leader and motivator of the research staff. The role also carries responsibility to supervise students registered for higher degrees (PhD, MPhil) and assist senior researchers to develop their supervisory skills, grant writing skills and national reputation. Beyond immediate research commitments the professor is required to participate in departmental and faculty research development and participate in national professional bodies/societies.

Lecturer

Within university departments lecturers are employed with a significant teaching responsibility however the department normally has a commitment to contribute to the overall research output of the university. This can be achieved in a number of ways, usually through dedicated scholarly activity; the physiotherapy lecturer may be

2.8

encouraged to complete a PhD and so pursue an area of individual interest. Many lecturers/senior lecturers manage masters' modules and have the opportunity to coordinate research projects and finally physiotherapy undergraduates may complete a research project supervised by a lecturer. To fulfil these research obligations a lecturer must have the skills to understand and supervise the research process as well as providing pastoral support for the students. A lecturer should be able to contribute and develop reports/publications to disseminate the findings.

Clinical researcher

A clinical researcher is usually based within a healthcare organisation and can also be a permanent post. Interestingly many of the higher clinical grades within the agenda for change schedule require there to be some research activity.

Physiotherapists can be employed to completely pre-defined clinical trials sponsored by a pharmaceutical or equipment company under strict guidance from the company funding the research. However, this is a very different role to an independent clinical researcher. This type of research role, while not developing an independent research project does allow an introduction to the rigours of measurement and data collection.

A clinical researcher often has a pre-defined commitment to research, often in the region of 50 per cent. The clinical researcher is both a clinical expert and an independent researcher. The research projects are usually embedded into a physiotherapy service, and meet all the requirements of the local ethics committee and conform to good clinical practice guidelines.

Research consultant

A research consultant, as implied is employed as a consultant to pre-defined research projects and time contributed to the project is costed accordingly. The consultant researcher has an established track record in the area of research and is acknowledged as an expert in that area. The skills required for this include excellent communication skills, writing skills and report writing. The clients may request that the consultant is involved in the dissemination of results and therefore excellent presentation skills are required to give information in a number of formats.

Research orientated manager

A research manager usually has one of two roles, either associated with a larger research department or specifically employed on a specific research project grant. The more general research managers are employed within NHS research and development (R&D) offices or within university research departments. An NHS research manager's primary responsibility is to ensure that any research activity has the necessary ethics committee and NHS R&D approval and the research staff on the project conform to good clinical practice (GCP) guidelines. Research managers are knowledgeable about research funding opportunities through research councils, charities and the National Institute for Health Research. Generally the role of a research manager is to assist in/ensure:
- safe and ethically responsible care.
- participant recruitment.
- advancing to code of ethics and institutional guidelines.
- annual/final research reports are written.
- financial monitoring meets the required standards.

If a research manager is employed to a specific project it is likely they will have additional responsibility for the recruitment process of staff to the project.

2.9 A junior contract researcher
Rupert Kerrell

Types of contract and their implications ~ scope of work ~ experience and skills needed ~ skills developed ~ options post-contract

Working as a junior contract researcher is highly rewarding and exciting. It can offer you the opportunity to continue working with a clinical focus, giving you the chance to develop new skills that can be used in the clinical setting (if you decide to return to clinical work) or it can provide you with a sound base to continue as a researcher.

Types of contracts and their implications

- Fixed or on-going
- Length of contract
- Title

Fixed or on-going
A contract may be a fixed term that is finishing after a specified time or on-going. An on-going contract may occur as the project evolves. In this case additional funding may be requested, and if successful, the project will continue.

Once you are working in a particular location there may be opportunities to work on different research projects once your original contract has ended.

Length of contract
As a junior contract researcher there are a number of options regarding the length of your employment. It could be a short-term contract lasting approximately six months or a longer contract (for more in-depth studies) lasting around three years.

Longer contracts for a single piece of work are unlikely although you may be working as a junior researcher while completing a PhD, in which case the contract could be longer.

Title
Often the funding for the project has been secured prior to your employment by a more senior researcher. Your title might therefore reflect that you are working for someone else so you maybe employed as a research assistant or research associate.

Scope of work

- Types of research
- Places to work
- Junior contract researcher role
- Further qualifications

Types of research
The type of research completed normally fits into one of two categories, qualitative or quantitative; however some research may contain a combination of the two. Bowling and Ebrahim (2007) describe qualitative methods as:
'the collection of narratives, interviews, focus groups.... which can provide rich insights into the experience of individuals, the meaning and interpretation of those experiences, and the likely relationships between different factors'. (p7).

Conversely quantitative methods have:
'hypotheses that are constructed and tested in experiments that take place in tightly controlled conditions, and outcomes are measured with high precision.'
Bowling and Ebrahim, 2007 (p6).

Whichever type of research is being completed they all involve the collecting of some data and this could be done in a number of ways including interview, questionnaire, measurement/instrumentation or observation.

Places to work
The places where you could work are varied, and include hospital settings such as physiotherapy departments, joint therapies departments (for example physiotherapy, occupational therapy and speech and language), clinical specialist areas, and so on. There may also be opportunities in other healthcare areas such as in the community, primary care trusts and GP surgeries.

You could also be employed by universities, within uni-professional or multi-professional settings (for example allied health professions departments). Within universities there could be vacancies within more specialised areas such as the biomechanics department, involving a laboratory-based setting.

2.9

The junior contract researcher role

When working as a junior contract researcher you may be involved in a wide range of studies. It may include collecting data from subjects for a more senior researcher; or it may, depending on your skills, involve analysing data that has already been collected, completing an audit within a hospital department or evaluating a particular aspect of treatment.

In most cases you will have a supervisor with overall responsibility for the project, who has a good grounding and knowledge of the research process and project management. They may also have a range of contacts for you to make use of if there are areas in which you need specialist skills or knowledge (for example statistics).

The amount of patient or client contact varies greatly between different projects, and is influenced by the type of project you are doing. For example, data collection via measurement probably involves more direct contact than analysing completed questionnaires.

Further qualifications

In some contracts there may be opportunities to gain further formal qualifications while working on the project, for example a masters degree, an MPhil or doctorate.

Experiences and skills needed

- Formal qualifications
- Previous experience

Formal qualifications

Many junior researcher jobs do not require any qualifications other than a pre-registration qualification (normally a BSc). However your options as a contract researcher could be increased if you have an MSc.

Completing a Masters degree develops skills useful to a researcher, such as the ability to critically appraise journal articles (useful when completing literature searches and reviews). A postgraduate degree should also provide you with an opportunity to complete a research project and therefore gain experience in, for example, considering ethical issues and gaining research governance approval, using different types of analysis and writing reports.

Previous experience
While there are junior research jobs that do not require an MSc, having some previous experience in any type of research or audit increases your understanding of the research process, and is very useful.

Prior to working as a junior researcher it is preferable that you have a sound clinical base. It is usual to have been working at Band 6 level (or equivalent) prior to starting, or to be in your first Band 6 job having worked clinically for at least 12 months.

Skills developed

- Informal skills
- Formal qualifications

There could be a number of reasons why you may want to work as a junior contract researcher: to experience another facet of physiotherapy professional life; to develop research skills; or to start a career in research and add to the evidence base for physiotherapy.

Informal skills
There are many skills that you will develop while working as a junior contract researcher which may be new to you. Such skills can have a direct benefit on your clinical work (if you return to that field) or be very useful as you continue your research career.

Although all physiotherapists and AHPs practise within a professional and ethical code of conduct, you now have to consider formally the ethical aspects of your research project. In the majority of cases this means completing an ethics application form and then submitting this to the hospital, university, local or regional ethics committee. In order to complete this form successfully you need to clearly demonstrate that a number of issues have been addressed. These include ensuring that: informed consent

2.9

is gained; participants will be protected at all stages of the project; discomfort for participants is minimised; privacy is maintained; and that it is clear who will actually benefit from the research being completed.

You new role may mean that, although you might be part of a bigger project team, you are in reality mainly working as a lone researcher. Working to deadlines and not on throughput (for example the number of patients you have seen) could be different from your previous clinical work. In a researcher role you have to meet targets and deadlines for the project (often set out in a Gantt chart: another skill you may acquire!). This often requires greater flexibility in your work patterns and schedule. You need to be self-disciplined and self-motivated: there are quieter periods, as well as busy periods, where to meet deadlines work needs to be completed in the evenings or at weekends.

There is normally an expectation that the results of the project need to be disseminated either via publication or presentation. By writing articles for publication you will develop your writing style. This differs, depending on the journal you are writing for. For example, writing a piece for *Frontline* is different from writing an article for *The Lancet* or *Physiotherapy*.

In order to present your findings at conferences successfully, you need to decide how and what to present. Many conferences offer opportunities to present papers, lead roundtable discussions, complete a poster, and so on. The skills needed for each of these are different and develop the more you present.

Formal qualifications

You may finish your time as a junior contract researcher with a formal qualification – this depends on what was agreed at the beginning of the contract. If, as part of the project, you have completed an MSc or PhD this is a formal recognition of your continuing professional development and may result in further career opportunities and, in some cases, better pay.

You may not have the opportunity (or inclination) to complete a PhD during the project in which case you there may be an opportunity to register for an MPhil which is a research degree, requiring the completion of a thesis.

After your junior researcher contract ends

Following your time as a junior researcher you may continue working in research, and with the skills you have developed you could take on more responsibility on other projects and/or prepare bids to secure funding for your own projects.

You may wish to return to clinical work, where you will be able to utilise the skills you have recently developed such as critical analysis, time management, working to deadlines and being able to find, digest and present pertinent information.

Summary

The short-term nature of this role gives you the chance to gain some research experience before fully committing to it for your future career. You get the opportunity to work with seasoned researchers and develop skills that can be used in a wide variety of health settings. Working as a junior contract researcher provides you with an ideal opportunity to either start your research career, or to see what it is really like to work in research.

References
- Bowling A, Ebrahim S. Handbook of Health Research Methods: investigation, measurement and analysis (2007) . Open University Press, Maidenhead.

2.10 A clinical researcher
Rhoda Allison

Role of the clinical researcher ~ opportunities for clinical research ~ conducting clinical research ~implementing clinical research ~ a personal experience of clinical research

Role of the clinical researcher

Clinical researchers are generally those conducting research into subjects directly related to clinical practice. Many of these individuals combine a role participating in research activity with responsibilities for clinical practice.

The advantages of combining the roles are significant. Frontline clinicians are well placed to pose appropriate and relevant questions for research and ensure it is grounded in reality and potential patient benefit. Equally, involvement of clinicians in research works to raise standards across clinical practice: there is a positive correlation between achievement of high ratings on the Healthcare Commission Quality Ratings (2006) and NHS organisations' involvement in research activity.

As academic institutions make closer links with healthcare providers, and with the development of Local Research Networks, there are more opportunities to combine roles and bring research activity directly into the workplace.

Opportunities for clinical research

All research needs to be adequately funded. This includes funding for researchers' time, clerical support and sundries. There are a number of potential sources of funding and support available to aspiring researchers:
- Links with academic partners.
- Research networks.
- Other grants.

Links with academic partners
It's probably fair to say that while academic institutions have access to staff skilled in research planning and design, providers of clinical services have access to specialised clinicians and the patient population. Therefore, partnerships between the two are advantageous to both, and aspiring researchers may find it useful to establish partnerships with local academic departments as a first step.

Research networks

In 2006 national research funding streams were reviewed and reallocated (DH, 2006). One consequence of this was the development of National Clinical Research Networks, which were built around improving research capacity in particular clinical areas such as cancer, diabetes and stroke. Each National Network supports a number of Local Research Networks which are funded to undertake research on nationally adopted studies. Ideas are generated or approved via Clinical Studies Groups and are then fed down to local level where local networks can choose which studies from a portfolio they participate in. The networks are usually partnerships between NHS organisations and Research Institutions, and their success is measured by rates of recruitment into clinical trials.

Development of local networks has led to the development of many more clinical research roles in NHS trusts which can potentially be full-time or part-time and thus combined with clinical roles. These include opportunities for novices as well as more experienced researchers, and networks can generate their own ideas and submit these for adoption to the Clinical Studies Groups. This has been a significant opportunity for front line healthcare staff to become engaged in nationally funded research projects.

Grants

Many charities linked to particular conditions such as Arthritis Care have research funds, although bids are very competitive and the reputation of the research team would be a major factor in allocating the funds. Some of these organisations offer particular funds to support Allied Health Professionals – for example the Stroke Association offers several bursaries for AHPs to undertake doctorate studies each year.

The Department of Health also offers Researcher Development Awards which have been secured by Allied Health Professionals for doctorate studies. These funds are contestable, so again the academic support available would be a factor in being a successful applicant.

The Research for Patient Benefit Programme is an NHS nationally co-ordinated funding stream for research commissioned on a regional basis. Each region receives funds based on size of population and allocates grants for research evaluating different interventions and methods of service delivery. The programme accepts applications several times each year.

In addition, there are still some funding streams for research outside the formal clinical research networks so there is still potential to apply to NHS R&D departments for support with projects.

2.10

Conducting clinical research

All NHS organisations follow research governance and ethical approval processes. If you work within the NHS your local research and development lead will be able to advise you of these processes. They may also be able to advise on other support available as being a lone researcher in a department can be quite an isolated role.

Implementing research

Although designing and conducting research is a skilful task, it would all be for nothing if good quality research findings are not used to change clinical practice. Systematic reviews can be used to develop clinical guidelines, although there are many areas for practice where there is insufficient quality evidence to guide this process and consensus among clinicians is still used to develop less robust evidence-based clinical guidance tools. Lead clinicians have a responsibility to review the best evidence and guidelines available and to ensure these are implemented in organisations. Clinical audit should be used to measure the success of these strategies.

A personal experience of clinical research

Since my first job as a junior physiotherapist I have been interested in the potential for conducting research in the clinical setting, as well as implementing research findings. However, my aspirations became more focused while working in New Zealand when I was fortunate to have a role as professional lead of an acute and community provider and was in a position to build relationships with local academic partners. Together we were successful in bidding for grants to be able to conduct fairly small projects evaluating interventions in the clinical setting.

After returning to the UK, I again sought out local academic partners and was able to work with staff from the local university conducting a small project to begin with, but then bidding for larger funds. Throughout this time, my job plan did not contain dedicated research time and it was a constant challenge to make time for this within a busy clinical role. However, we worked with the local university to set up a funded project where one of our clinicians has funding for research one day per week for a specific project.

I became a consultant physiotherapist three years ago and now have dedicated research time within my job plan. We have conducted pilot projects comparing interventions in stroke, and I applied for a small grant from the Primary Care Research Network which helped fund a project on secondary prevention of stroke but more importantly introduced me to the Primary Care Division of the local Medical School. They were able to support me with the project and we are now involved in discussions about potential for further research. I am the Rehabilitation Lead for the Peninsular Local Research Network and have worked with the steering group to ensure we have a balance selection of studies including some with rehabilitation focus as well as acute.

Throughout my career my time spent on research has always been much less than my time in clinical practice and it's always a challenge to balance the two. There are real benefits however and I enjoy the ability to work across both. For clinicians who do not have dedicated research time, the responsibility for implementing research findings can not be overlooked. The CSP produce a number of evidence-based products as do many condition focused groups such as the Intercollegiate Working Party for Stroke. Implementation and audit of clinical guidelines or direct research findings is just as important as actually conducting research.

Reflecting on my own experience, there are two key messages I would give to any aspiring clinical researcher. First, that everything takes much more time than you imagine. This applies to every part of the process, so you need to be realistic about what you will achieve. Second, the value of developing partnerships is essential to conducting clinical research, and if this is your interest I would recommend seeking out either local champions within your own organisation or in academic organisations who can support you.

Reference list
- Department of Health. Best Research for Best Health. A New National Health Research Strategy. (2006). The NHS contribution to health research in England: a consultation. DOH London.

- Healthcare Commission. Results of the annual health check 2005/2006. (2006). Healthcare Commission, London.

2.11 An experienced researcher
Nadine E Foster

Developing your research path beyond initial research training ~ following that research path as an experienced researcher ~ developing as a research leader ~ example ~ a final note

An 'experienced researcher' in physiotherapy is not simple to define. It is probably better to view the development of research experience as a continuum, rather than to focus on any single definition. At one end of the continuum is the early career researcher who has just completed their initial research training, for example a PhD. At the other end is the research leader, who has the skills, track record, experience and vision to lead an active group of researchers capable of competing at national and international levels of research. An experienced researcher is a potential future research leader, although clearly not all experienced researchers will progress in this way. This chapter summarises key challenges in, and recommendations for, the development of a career as an experienced researcher.

Developing your research path beyond initial research training

Once you have obtained your research training through, for example, a PhD programme, you are likely to have developed expertise in a reasonably narrow topic area and/or research methodology. In order to progress as a researcher, you will need to develop your own research path beyond this initial research training.

There are different challenges at each stage of a research career. While there is no single ideal approach in developing a research path to become an experienced researcher, this is most likely to require a degree of flexibility about your topic area and/or research methodologies. Some of the most successful experienced researchers are those who, while retaining and further developing their original topic area, proceed to:
- broaden their expertise to fit with institutional, national and international research priorities.
- develop or work with strong collaborative teams, comprising individuals with different but complementary expertise and skills.
- invest considerable time and energy in developing research capacity and capability in others so that, over time, they build and support a critical mass of more junior researchers to support their research programmes.

One of the most critical points in your career path, determining whether and how you will progress as an experienced researcher, is the postdoctoral period. A major concern is that although there are increasing numbers of physiotherapists completing research degrees, few go on to develop as experienced researchers, capable of competing in research at national and international level with colleagues from other disciplines. There are many potential reasons for this, including the historical lack of specific postdoctoral funding opportunities and the unfortunate inflexibility of many physiotherapy careers in the past. In order to increase the chances of a positive postdoctoral period, or equivalent, that will support you to develop as an experienced researcher:

- actively seek working environments that support your research development.
- secure support and mentorship from more experienced researchers, either within or outside of your own research area or discipline, that can provide you with not only research guidance but also sound advice on career planning.
- if you do not have a supportive environment at your place of work, seek that support through individuals or networks externally and/or seriously consider moving to a more supportive environment.
- actively seek out established, or build new, collaborative networks for your research. Include those who are more experienced in your field and whose track record in publication and successful grant application can serve to both inspire and challenge you.
- apply for dedicated postdoctoral or equivalent funding, to support you to develop your expertise and skills further. Be prepared for several knock-backs in that process.
- view the years following your initial research training or research degree as a period of consolidation and growth and seek out opportunities that will deepen your expertise. Not all of these activities will be positive, or lead to worthwhile research avenues or collaborations, but many will, and may provide important learning experiences.

Following that research path as an experienced researcher

There are many different examples of career paths that result in physiotherapists working in experienced research roles: within academia, clinical settings, industry or a combination of these. Increased flexibility and specific funding for opportunities to combine research with clinical and/or educational roles is likely to support a growing cadre of physiotherapists to develop as experienced researchers, as well as ensure that

2.11

the research is relevant to and embedded within practice. In addition to building on the previous suggestions for the postdoctoral or equivalent period, more experienced researchers are likely to:
- demonstrate a broadening of research expertise across related topic areas and research methodologies.
- focus on a small number of areas of key expertise, yet also be sufficiently flexible to fit with research group, institutional, national and international research priorities.
- develop or work with strong collaborative teams comprising individuals with different but complementary expertise and skills, such as clinical specialties, health services research, health economics and statistics.
- demonstrate increasing project management skills that ensure the research is successfully delivered within the available resources.
- develop research capacity and capability in others, including guiding more junior research staff, such as postdoctoral physiotherapists, in their career development.
- develop and support research programmes rather than discrete research projects.
- meet the universal expectations of research excellence, including those of research publications, successful grant applications and supervision of research students and staff.
- understand that considerable breadth of experience is needed to be competitive at national and international levels, particularly in gaining the most competitive research funding.
- contribute increasingly to external research initiatives, reviewing others' research and becoming involved in funding committees and other research decision-making bodies.

One of the key challenges faced by those who have developed successful records of research achievement, is the risk of increasing levels of administrative workload that serve to constrain and diminish further research achievement and excellence. Key actions that can support the experienced researcher through these challenges include:
- securing further career development funding, in addition to programme and project specific funding, that protects the experienced researcher's time for focused research activity.
- careful career planning and guidance, including the contribution of respected mentor(s) and formal research leadership training.
- working within a unit or group with sufficient infrastructure support, so that the administrative burden can be minimised and time protected for grant writing, publication and research activities.

Developing as a research leader

The goal of some experienced researchers in physiotherapy will be to progress as research leaders. They will build research teams that are capable of success in the delivery of research programmes, as required by the demands of national and international competition. While there are many different routes to increasing your levels of autonomy and independence and becoming a research leader, there are a number of common attributes:
- a clear and long-term contribution to research development and capacity in a chosen field.
- an increasing role in the strategic decisions about the research programmes to which different research teams contribute.
- an increasing responsibility for the overall quality of research programmes and the contribution they make, including responding to external quality assessment activities.
- an increasing accountability for the direction and financial support of research programmes and associated research staff to their institutions and funding bodies.
- an increasing accountability for the 'fit' of the research group's activity with institutional research ambitions and resources.
- the leadership of teams comprising varied professional backgrounds and areas of expertise, including contract research staff, postgraduate research students and administrative and support staff.
- a nationally or internationally recognised research record and a clear research vision that can inspire and challenge more junior staff.

Example

My research career was inspired by a positive experience as an undergraduate physiotherapist, when I was able to conduct a small but clinically based research project. From there, I combined a small clinical workload alongside a doctoral programme of research within a supportive research environment, enriched by colleagues across different research disciplines and experiences. My early postdoctoral years were spent gaining experience in education and administration combined with developing my research depth and breadth. This included building research collaborations in different directions: some of these were short-lived but others continue to thrive. Supervising and developing others in research has been, and still is, a particularly rewarding experience.

2.11

My current post is based within a dedicated university research centre, funded through a Department of Health Career Scientist Award managed by the National Co-ordinating Centre for Research Capacity Development (NCCRCD), now replaced by the NIHR Senior Research Fellowship. I have five years of funding to deliver a programme of research and develop research teams and collaborative partnerships within the programme. I am a principal investigator for this research programme and for several projects, leading the research teams within each. My role includes securing new grant income to support and extend the research activity, including funding for the staff employed in research posts, liaising with stakeholders including clinicians, NHS trust managers and patients, and contributing to the strategic decisions about the future of the research programmes to fit with institutional priorities and agendas.

Maintaining and developing my own research expertise and publication track record is a continuing priority, alongside a small teaching and administrative workload. I have a key role in the supervision of more junior researchers from a range of clinical and non-clinical backgrounds. This includes the full range of research activities from protocol development, ethical and research approvals, project management and completion, presentation and publication, grant writing, reviewing and supervision. An important part of my current role involves research team building and management, developing research capacity and collaborations, and attracting significant further research funding. External activities include involvement in research and professional societies, organising conferences, grant and research paper reviewing and making decisions about research funding through committee memberships nationally and internationally.

A final note

It is worth viewing a research career in physiotherapy as just that, a full and long-term career. For those who enter a research career early and go on to develop as an experienced researcher, this can mean more or less a whole working life of research activity and experience. Seeing the big picture will help to motivate you in those times when rejected papers or grant applications, or other negative experiences, drain your enthusiasm and threaten your tenacity. Time and effort in building particularly good postdoctoral experience will provide you with a range of skills and experiences to draw on, and will help you meet the demands of a role as an experienced researcher.

Further information
- There are courses available on research team leadership, such as those from the Leadership Foundation for Higher Education, see **www.lfue.ac.uk/support/rtl/** and courses on leadership in general that can support your own personal and career development, such as those from the King's Fund, see **www.kingsfund.org.uk/leadership/index.html**
- There are online resources to support the leadership development of principal investigators. For example, see **www.le.ac.uk/researchleader/**
- Research Excellence Framework. See **www.hefce.ac.uk/research/assessment/reform**
- Funding to support postdoctoral programmes and career research programmes are increasingly available. For example, the National Institute for Health Research (NIHR) offers postdoctoral fellowships, career development fellowships and senior research fellowships, see **www.nccrcd.nhs.uk/nihrfellow**
- For information about the UK Clinical Research Collaborations initiative on 'Developing the best research professionals' see **www.ukcrc.org/activities/researchworkforce.aspx**

2.12 A Lecturer
Lorna Paul

Introduction ~ opportunities for lecturers to be involved in research ~ university perspective on lecturers' involvement in research ~ challenges for lecturers being 'research active' ~ conclusion

Introduction

Although research is not always explicitly stated in the main roles and remits of a lecturer it is highly embedded and implicit within the role. Lecturers are involved in research at a number of different levels: from using research evidence to underpin teaching, through to leading large scale multicentre trials. This chapter will discuss how lecturers interact with the research process and what opportunities and challenges are faced by lecturers in undertaking research.

Opportunities for lecturers to be involved in research

Physiotherapy prides itself on, wherever possible, delivering services which are of high quality and evidence-based. When teaching students, whether undergraduate or postgraduate, the theory and practice delivered must be current and evidence-based. This means the lecturer must have a good critical understanding of the research process and be able to apply that knowledge to the teaching in their own specialised area, e.g. paediatrics, women's health. The lecturer must therefore have a firm understanding of literature searching, systems of critical appraisal, the levels of evidence, the process of undertaking and publishing a systematic review, the formation, limitations, implementation and evaluation of evidence-based guidelines, the different sources of guidelines, the concepts of clinical effectiveness, clinical governance and the national service frameworks. Thus, while some lecturers may not necessarily be actively involved in research projects, they must have a firm grounding in the research process and the use of research in clinical practice.

At another level, lecturers are generally involved in the supervision of student projects and dissertations. In a well-organised department, the expectation would be that the lecturer would propose a number of student projects that are aligned to their own research interests. This is mutually beneficial for both the student and supervisor for three main reasons: first, the student can undertake a project that may be laboratory-based but with a clinical application; second, the student should have a better supervisory experience, as the supervisor knows the topic and is better able to guide and support the student; and third, the supervisor may obtain some useful data with the student. This might, for example, be used as pilot data for a larger study, for publication in a peer reviewed journal or be submitted as a conference abstract. Thus, although the lecturer might not be carrying out the project personally, they must have a good understanding of it and sufficient research skills to supervise the student undertaking the project. A well conducted piece of student research not only benefits the student, perhaps encouraging them to consider research as part of their future career, but it may also enhance the research portfolio of the supervisor and ultimately the profile of the host university and the student's workplace.

Lecturers may also be studying towards a higher degree or, depending on the level of expertise of the lecturer, they may be involved in the supervision of students studying towards a PhD or even postdoctoral research assistants or fellows. The number of physiotherapists with, or studying towards, a PhD is steadily increasing. PhD students undertake a larger scale research project which must make some original contribution to the existing knowledge in the chosen specialist area. A PhD takes a minimum of three years (full-time) to complete, and as such, represents a significant commitment of time and effort by both the student, and their supervisor(s). Supervising PhD students can be a very satisfying experience: the lecturer sees their student growing in skills and confidence over the course of their study. The reverse, of course, can also be true if the close relationship between PhD student and supervisor becomes fraught and difficult, although the latter situation tends to be the exception rather than the norm.

So lecturers are involved in using research and research findings to underpin their teaching and they supervise students undertaking research projects at both undergraduate and postgraduate levels. Many lecturers also have personal research interests which they wish to pursue. Universities, often referred to as higher education institutions (HEIs), usually have good infrastructure in place to help support and develop lecturers undertaking research.

Generally within a university setting there is an established research hierarchy in place from vice-principals to deans and senior professors. These senior researchers have the experience and expertise to support, supervise and/or mentor more novice researchers such as lecturers. The diversity of staff within universities means expertise may be available in a range of research methodologies, both qualitative and quantitative. There may be good opportunity for inter- or cross-disciplinary collaboration, for example with other allied health care professionals, or other professional groups, such as those with expertise in computing. Statistical and health economics support may also be available within the HEIs. In terms of facilities, HEIs generally have good computing and library facilities and may have other specialised facilities such as movement laboratories. In economic terms, being part of an academic department may open up research funding opportunities both internal and external to the university, and fee waivers are often available for academic staff undertaking higher degrees such as PhDs.

University perspective on lecturers' involvement in research

Universities use the term 'research active' to describe academic staff who, as the name suggests, are actively involved in research! In real terms this means someone who is publishing research papers, supervising PhD students and securing grant income to undertake research. It is critically important for universities to have a high percentage of 'research active' academic staff and research generally features quite highly within the mission statements of most universities. University departments are set targets

TABLE 1

Examples of performance indicators for research

Academic papers published – • Number of papers • Impact factor of Journal	Postgraduate students • Number • Funding source – external or internal
Grant income • Total amount • Full economic cost recovery • Source – charity, funding councils, commercial	Percentage of staff who are research active in terms of • Publications • Grants • Postgraduate student supervision
Conference papers • Keynote address • National and international	Other esteem indicators • Membership of national/international committees • Membership of grant awarding panels • Journal editor or membership of editorial boards

or key performance indicators (KPIs) which are aligned to the university mission statement. There are targets for many areas of academic performance such as the quality of teaching and the student experience, and metrics will be developed in relation to the KPIs on which the department will report its research activity. There are a number of different metrics; however, some possible components are shown in Table 1.

Universities also strive to show success in the Research Assessment Exercise (RAE), soon to become the Research Excellence Framework (REF). The RAE is conducted jointly by the Higher Education Funding Councils of England, Scotland, Wales and the Department for Employment and Learning in Northern Ireland. The format of the RAE changes with each assessment exercise, but generally involves HEIs submitting a report of their research, in a specific format, to a discipline-based external panel for review. Through this process a grade is awarded, and depending on the grade, additional funding may be obtained. The most recent RAE occurred in 2008 and the metrics used for judging the quality of each submission were similar to those reported in Table 1, although the research environment, support and facilities were also considered.

Challenges for lecturers in being 'research active'

While there are increasing opportunities for lecturers to become involved in research there are, unsurprisingly, challenges as well. The main barrier to lecturers being involved in research is the old enemy time! As would be expected from the title of the post, the main roles and remits of a Lecturer are concerned with teaching. Thus the primary focus is preparing material and teaching at undergraduate and postgraduate level. Other roles and remits, however, will include development and delivery of continuing professional development courses, setting and marking student assessments, student advice and pastoral support, clinical visits and supervision, course or module leadership, coordination roles, meetings and committee membership. In addition there will probably be a time limited requirement to complete a formal teaching qualification to at least postgraduate certificate level. Issues such as staffing levels and staff/student ratios also have an impact on the amount of time possible for research. Some universities are known to place more emphasis on their research output and as such have strategies in place to allow staff more time for research activities. In comparison, other universities, tend to be more teaching focused.

2.12

There may be other challenges facing lecturers involved in research, for example if the research interests of a lecturer are not congruent with the research themes within the department or faculty. Table 2 provides a summary of possible barriers and drivers to a lecturer's involvement with research.

TABLE 2

Examples of drivers and barriers to lecturers being involved in research

DRIVERS	BARRIERS
Personal attributes • Self motivation and drive • Career progression • Need to add to professional evidence base • Would like to register for PhD	Personal attributes • Lack of interest or ideas • Lack of research skills • Scepticism • Lack of knowledge of current clinical problems • Lack of a PhD
Departmental issues • Good support for research including mentoring, resources • Research issues included in Personal Performance Review • Quality Enhancement University issues • Research Assessment Exercise • Opportunities for collaboration	Departmental issues • Lack of time • High teaching and administrative workload • Lack of resources • Poor research infrastructure • Research interests not congruent with current research themes University issues • Physiotherapy often in teaching focused institutions
Other factors • Funding opportunities • Political and social drivers and policy documents	Other factors • Personal life and interests • Difficulty in obtaining external funding especially as a novice researcher

Conclusion

So what drives those of us who are, or have been lecturers, to work long into the night to hit the deadline for a research grant application or to finalise the abstract for a conference, or a paper for publication? It is difficult to say definitively, but we have all done it on a regular basis. It may be the drive for future promotion within the research field, or it may be peer pressure from others in the research team to hit the deadlines! More probably the motivation comes from the buzz when the first data comes through on a project, from seeing your paper in print, from receiving the letter of award for your grant application or the acknowledgement of the contribution of your paper or work to the formation of a systematic review or guideline. Ultimately the motivation and drive is the realisation that your work has, to a greater or lesser extent, added to the evidence base which in the end will benefit the patient, client or carer.

Further information
- Research Assessment Exercise: **http://www.rae.ac.uk/**

2.13 A researching consultant
Laura Finucane

The four functions of the consultant role ~ expert clinical practice ~ professional leadership ~ education and professional development ~ practice and service development, research and evaluation ~ examples of how consultants influence clinical practice through the use of evidence

The Allied Health Professional (AHP) consultant came into existence in 2000 as part of the NHS Plan: *'New Consultant posts will provide better outcomes for patients, by retaining clinical excellence within the service.'* (DH, 2000)

This new role recognises the contribution that AHP's make to the healthcare of the nation. The role was developed to drive the NHS plan by redesigning services and developing protocols for service development. There are four inter-related functions that underpin the consultant role, and clinical expertise is at the core.

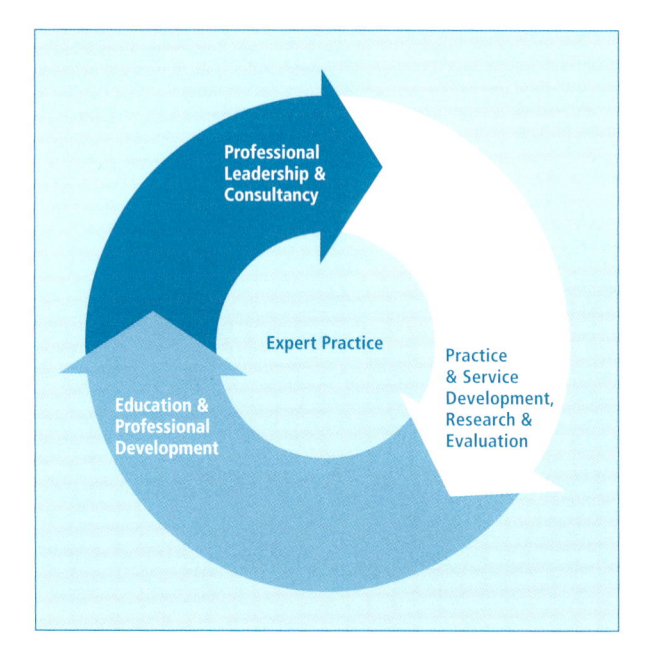

Until recently, therapists wanting to stay in a clinically-focused role in the NHS were unable to do so and often ended up in managerial posts. This resulted in a loss of clinical expertise (van Griensven, 2007). The development of consultants, clinical specialists and extended scope practitioners has ensured a much needed clinical pathway.

The four functions of the consultant role

Expert clinical practice
This is achieved by the consultant's continuation as a clinical expert and the implementation of evidence-based best practice. One of the main roles for a consultant is to act as a clinical champion within their field. Their responsibility is to deliver a whole-system, patient-focused approach through best practice. The creation of protocols of care, and design of care pathways through an evidence base, is an integral part of the role.

Professional leadership (supporting function)
The consultant is an effective leader who can challenge current structures, leading to the development of strategic plans: ultimately they can drive change and redesign services. The role provides expert opinion, based on best practice at trust level, in order to influence and deliver the clinical governance agenda.

Education and professional development (supporting function)
The role helps to facilitate the development of individuals' continuing professional development, by providing an environment that supports learning. The consultant acts as a mentor. In some cases the consultant teaches at Higher Education Institutions (HEIs) in their given field and may lecture or publish research in professional journals. The consultant is responsible for facilitating others to reach their full potential, providing an environment which promotes a learning culture within the organisation.

Practice and service development, research and evaluation (supporting function)
The role of the consultant is to ensure that services are based on the best available evidence.

Consultants are well placed to undertake and facilitate research that can enhance the evidence base by identifying where further research is needed. All consultants demonstrate masters level knowledge as a minimum requirement, with some having completed doctorates or being in the process of doing so. There is a strong role in developing partnerships with HEIs.

2.13

Although the consultant is expected to demonstrate competencies within each of these areas, the weighting will vary from post to post and in the main this is driven by local needs (Stevenson, 2003). The role of researcher may not be one of the strongest elements in many posts, yet it probably underpins all the roles the consultant is expected to fulfil. For example, a clinical expert requires a knowledge base of best practice and best evidence. It also requires the ability to challenge current thinking and evaluate the evidence base through further research, and to interpret and disseminate national guidelines to others in a meaningful way to enhance practice at all levels.

There are a number of posts that have protected time allocated to research activity. This may be because the post has been developed in conjunction with universities who contribute financially to the post and consequently have control over the amount of time allocated for research. These posts are few and far between but are nonetheless important and valuable in contributing to the body of knowledge.

However, the majority of posts are not able to spend time researching as this is not the main function of the post. Although there is probably an expectation on the part of managers that the consultant carries out research in some capacity, it is not necessarily supported in terms of designated time. It is perhaps sometimes perceived as a low priority for the role. This tends not to be the opinion of the consultants themselves, who feel their contribution to research is important, however small. Research is not just about clinical trials: contributions to the body of research can be achieved in many different ways. A considerable number of clinicians are undertaking higher level degrees, and the consultant has the opportunity to influence areas of research at this level. Support through development of ideas and mentorship of research projects are an integral aspect of the role, and can help to develop services and ultimately to enhance practice. For example, they might evaluate a new outcome tool that screens patients, ensuring they receive the appropriate treatment in a timely manner.

A number of consultants have been involved in the development of a broad range of national guidelines, such as those for Parkinson's disease and low back pain, or the Musculoskeletal Service Framework (DoH 2006). The contribution to professional guidelines and protocols of care ensure that therapists have a voice and representation (Keilty and Bott, 2006). The current government 18-week pathway target has substantial implications for the delivery of musculoskeletal services. At a national level there is representation by a consultant, who provides expert opinion to the DoH in the development of pathways. At a local level, consultants are influencing pathways to ensure that the best practice is at the heart of these targets. This expert opinion is based on knowledge of best practice.

Examples of how consultants influence clinical practice through the use of evidence

Evidence-based practice is a core part of any therapist's role. One of the roles of the consultant is to continually evaluate and challenge the evidence and interpret its meaning, while facilitating practitioners' appropriate use of the evidence.

In 2003 a consultant physiotherapist set up a Clinically Appraised Topics group (CATS) in response to questions posed by clinicians. The idea was to be able to answer questions that come up on a daily basis. Issues posed, such as the use of eccentric versus concentric exercises in Achilles tendonopathies, were evaluated through literature searches and appraisal of the evidence. The research appraisal was conducted by clinicians. This innovative practice has encouraged clinicians to evaluate the evidence and transfer it into practice. Clinicians involved in the group felt their appraisal skills had been enhanced and they were able to influence their everyday practice.

My own personal experience of fulfilling the research function of the post has been challenging. The current priority to meet local health needs has meant that a formal research component has not always been possible. Because I recognise the importance of having some research involvement, I felt I wanted to undertake it in some capacity. Part of the skill of a consultant is having the ability to incorporate it, despite having an abundance of other commitments.

My current activity involves the interpretation of national guidelines such as those on low back pain and whiplash, making it meaningful for staff at a clinical level. Postgraduate courses are partly funded through the trust, and I support postgraduate students in a clinical capacity and with their masters dissertations. This has allowed application to practice by identifying areas of research that would benefit the needs of the local economy, as well as adding to the evidence base.

My involvement with the South East Musculoskeletal Research and Audit Clinical Academic Collaborative group has contributed to my role. The purpose of the group is to work in collaboration with other hospitals at a clinical level to address topical issues. It provides a forum for clinicians to be active in research and to present their audits in a supportive environment. This has helped to develop a research culture and identify areas that are both important

2.13

clinically and locally to the health economy. In the context of this group, I have personally been involved in a research project evaluating the incidence of sinister spinal pathologies. It is rewarding that this piece of work will be presented as a research paper at an international conference and a paper submitted to a professional journal.

At a national level I am a member of the executive committee for the Manipulative Association of the Chartered Physiotherapists (MACP). The MACP contributes to numerous governmental consultations regarding the future of research in the NHS, specifically in relation to Allied Health Professionals, and to proposed changes in the way ethical approval for research is sought. The MACP is also actively involved in the National Physiotherapy Research Network and the CSP Physiotherapy Guideline Programme review.

The MACP financially supports the undertaking and dissemination of research at all levels encouraging members to be involved with research.

My affiliation to the University of Brighton as a visiting fellow means that a clinical academic partnership has been developed and there is the potential to explore collaborative work. It is also an opportunity to support valuable research, through activities such as data collection.

Despite the time challenges and funding for this function, the role of research is clearly a subject that encompasses all areas of any consultant's post. Achieving this role as a researcher practitioner is not always easy, with many other aspects of the role taking priority particularly in this time of change. Despite these challenges the importance of research is strongly recognised within the consultant role. The ability to be flexible and creative with the time available will help to influence research at many different levels, which can be extremely rewarding.

Reference list
- Department of Health. Meeting the challenge: a strategy for allied health professions (2000).
- Department of Health. (2006). Musculoskeletal Service Framework.
- Keilty SEJ, Bott J. Opportunities in acute and chronic respiratory physiotherapy: Recent developments in the UK. Physical Therapy Reviews 11:44-48 (2006).

- Stevenson K. A New Dawn: A consultant physiotherapist in musculoskeletal disease. Musculoskeletal Care. 1 1 65-70 (2003).
- Van Griensven H. Consultant Physiotherapists - What's in a name? Primary care Today, 8 March/April (2007). **www.primarycaretoday.co.uk**

Further information
- The Chartered Society of Physiotherapy. Physiotherapy Consultant (NHS): Role, Attributes and guidance for establishing posts. PA56 (2002).

2.14 Leading clinical research
Jeremy Lewis

The purpose of clinical research ~ how to determine if clinical research is necessary ~ evidence-based practice ~ implementing a clinical research programme ~ developing a research programme ~ staging clinical research ~ research and ethics committees ~ funding ~ the clinical research cycle ~ translating clinical research

Clinical research

The purpose of clinical research
The primary aim of clinical research programmes is typically to find methods of improving the quality of healthcare that can be offered to individual patients within the local health environment. This can then inform the wider national and international healthcare communities so that the findings, if relevant, may be translated into their healthcare communities. Clinical research has the power to improve the health of individuals and societies. Without clinical research, we wouldn't know that smoking has a devastating effect on health, or that heart disease and nutrition are linked or that bed rest is inappropriate for mechanical back pain.

How to determine if clinical research is necessary
At a clinical level the most robust method of determining if research is required is to review and critically appraise the available and existing body of research knowledge in a specific area of clinical practice. This is to determine if the available information can guide clinical practice in a vigorous and meaningful manner, and relates both to the assessment and management of specific conditions. If the available evidence does not provide the information to direct clinical practice, then clinical research is not only necessary but obligatory.

At a personal level you only need to ask the following question to determine if clinical research is required: 'Would I be happy if [insert the name of someone you love or care for] had this outcome following this treatment?' if your answer is 'no' then on-going research is required.

Evidence-based practice
Our aim must be to develop better methods of assessment and management through a variety of research approaches. However, we must also acknowledge that the current body of research knowledge is not complete, and it would be inappropriate to discard areas of clinical practice because of a lack of evidence, unless the available evidence or experience suggested that the practice in question may be detrimental to an individual.

Clinical practice therefore should be based on the best available research evidence, the knowledge and experience of the clinician, the wishes, desires and beliefs of the patients, and the economic consequences of the practice. As our research knowledge grows this information may be used to better educate clinicians, healthcare communities, society and individual patients, and as a result our clinical practice, over time, will change.

Leading clinical research

Implementing a clinical research programme
In conjunction with other relevant individuals and groups it is the responsibility of the individual leading a programme of research to implement a relevant and sustainable clinical research programme. It is impossible to do everything all at once and it is therefore necessary to develop a graduated programme that takes into account all the available resources including: the strengths and weaknesses of all the individuals that will be involved; time; funding; equipment; management and organisational requirements; appropriate research patients; and research priorities. Those leading clinical research may be responsible for research within a specialty, sub-specialty, multi-disciplinary department, or research across a number of professions, organisations or countries.

Developing a research programme
It is essential for all relevant individuals and groups to meet to determine:
- Is there a need for clinical research?
- Is there a desire to proceed with research?
- What is the main purpose of the planned research?
- what are the potential benefits of the planned research?
- Are there sufficient resources for the research?
- What are the research priorities, how can they be achieved and in what order?
- Is it necessary to work collaboratively with others in the organisation, and how can this be achieved?
- Is it necessary to collaborate with others nationally and/or internationally and how can this be achieved?

After these decisions have been made and a research plan decided upon it is essential that a robust critical appraisal of the available research evidence and grey literature is performed to fully inform the research procedure. Before embarking on any clinical study it is crucial to review the existing research to identify what level of evidence is currently available and where deficiencies exist. Although not always possible, this review

2.14

process ideally should take the form of a systematic review. When a deficiency has been identified, a clinical research programme can be instigated.

Staging clinical research

Clinical research should build on existing knowledge or clinical beliefs, and may progress through many stages depending on the available resources and level of pre-existing knowledge. These stages may include: single case studies, case series, cohort studies and randomised controlled trails. Clinical studies may also involve determining the reliability and validity of clinical assessment procedures. Frequently pilot or preparatory studies need to be conducted before the larger more definitive study. These preparatory studies help to identify the feasibility of the larger study including the method of conducting the final study. Pilot studies are performed to investigate the reliability and amount of error associated with the measurement methods that will be used in the definitive study. Additionally these studies help to inform the research team how many subjects will need to be recruited into the final study. It is important that the research lead determines the research priorities and sequence to devise a strategy following discussion with those involved in the investigations.

Research and ethics committees

No research should proceed unless it has been peer-reviewed locally and by independent national and possibly international experts in the field. Ideally user involvement will form part of the review process to gain insight into how the relevant users of the research (patients, clinicians, health groups and agencies) perceive the proposal and potential outcomes. Formal submission to the local, regional or national research and development and ethics committees is mandatory. Their advice and guidance may be sought in preparing the research. It is the responsibility of the research lead to ensure that all the appropriate stages and milestones including appropriate training, submission, reviews, changes to the research protocol and understanding of the legal requirements of research have been complied with.

Funding

In the majority of cases research cannot progress unless adequate funding is secured. Funding is available from a variety of sources depending on the type of clinical research being planned. Costing a study can be very complicated and the guidance of healthcare economists, advisors and accountants is often required. This is to be certain that all the direct and obvious, and less obvious costs of a specific study or programme of research are accounted for. To participate in clinical studies clinicians generally require time to: conceptualise the investigation, perform a robust review of the literature, apply for grants, prepare and submit the study to ethics, participate in pre-project and research training programmes, perform the activities required of the investigation, analyse the data, write up the investigation and disseminate the findings. All these activities generally involve a loss of normal clinical time. This loss needs to be factored into the grant application so that a locum therapist or short-term contract position can be paid for so there is no real loss of clinical time as a result of the investigation. Another responsibility of the research lead is too identify appropriate sources of funding for specific investigations, write grant applications, support and guide others in writing their own grant applications, and identify groups to collaborate with in developing a grant application for a stand alone study or a programme of research. A research account will need to be set up with safeguards to ensure funds are spent appropriately and that the research remains within its set budget.

The clinical research cycle
When developing a clinical research programme the research leader will ideally have established a short, medium and long-term plan that identifies the investigations that will be conducted (i) locally (within and across departments), (ii) regionally and nationally, and (iii) internationally. One component of the research will be used to inform the next stage and the cycle will continue adding to the body of knowledge required to inform and improve clinical practice.

Translating clinical research
An essential role for the research leader is to ensure that the findings of clinical research are disseminated locally and, if appropriate, nationally and internationally. There are many ways that research may be disseminated. Often this is the hardest stage of the research cycle, as implementing change is very complicated and fraught with difficulty: it requires a chapter dedicated just to this issue. To demonstrate the difficulty of this stage is actually quite simple. We already know that a certain amount of physical exercise per week is very beneficial to a number of systems in the body as well as for psychological health. Published research in the areas of nutrition and weight control, smoking, and balancing work and leisure, attests to the potential for substantial improvements in the health of individuals and societies. There is little evidence that these relatively simple messages have been disseminated and implemented robustly. Therefore disseminating and implementing the findings of clinical research is a responsibility for everyone involved in the research process.

2.15 A research-oriented manager
Fiona Ottewell

The benefits of research to the manager ~ a research-orientated culture - facilitating staff involvement in audit projects or journal clubs ~ being responsible for a team of research therapists ~ how to sustain capacity for research ~ how to support the research practitioner

Does evidence-based practice (EBP) mean better care for patients?

Does the existence of research necessarily result in better care for patients? There is little data to indicate that the answer to this is 'yes'. In fact, there is more data suggesting that research evidence is often known, yet commonly ignored (Cochrane, 1976). However, for every pathway or protocol that has been drawn up, there will have been a piece of work examining the evidence to support that practice. Given that the protocols/pathways will have been drawn up to improve or streamline services this, at its most basic, will have improved patient care.

What is in it for me as a manager?

A manager or team leader has to be able to find a balance between quality and quantity of care. Robust evidence to support the best quality of care usually demonstrates the most effective use of resources in the long run. The team leader that harnesses this evidence can ensure a combination of effectiveness and efficiency (Porter and Teisberg, 2006). Using best practice should also result in increased productivity.

A manager has to be able to ensure that the various clinical governance requirements that exist in the healthcare environment of the 21st century are met in full. If research capacity is carefully managed, meeting the needs of your organisation's clinical governance programme becomes part of the daily business of your department. The facilitation of a research culture in which teams search and learn together is also a significant recruitment and retention tool (Borrill et al, 2001; West et al, 2002).

What will the research-orientated manager look for in therapists?

An existing or aspiring member of staff must be enthusiastic about research and use references in their presentations and at interview. They should also be aware of any research publications by interview panel members or key stakeholders, and understand what the key research issues are for the therapy team.

How to support research in the clinical environment

There are many ways in which research can be promoted within the clinical environment. The suggestions below will all potentially help research become part of the therapy team's culture and help to withstand the call for efficiencies and cost improvements:
- **Protected time:** set a standard for protected time for continuing professional development (CPD), including for research. This will be valuable even if it is not met 100 per cent of the time;
- **Audit:** set a robust audit programme. This should be led by senior staff and undertaken by assistants and rotational staff, as well as senior colleagues;
- **Projects (PDSA):** many audit or change projects have the potential to become action research projects;
- **Masters projects:** clinical leadership within therapy teams is important. The research-orientated manager should plan to have at least 1 per cent of their staffing resource undergoing masters training every three years;
- **Use of EBP roles:** identify senior staff for these roles and designate 30 per cent of their work time to evidence-based practice.

Cost-free Continuing Professional Development and publishing opportunities

- **Cochrane collaboration:** encourage staff who have completed masters degrees to retain their skills by participating in Cochrane reviews. This is free CPD (other than the time required) and your department may even get some backfill for the time;
- **Systematic reviews of the literature:** allied health professional bodies will periodically call for volunteers to participate in a review of the evidence. This is a wonderful opportunity for staff to network and receive freshly published evidence, and will ensure that your department is up-to-date with best practice;
- **Clinical supervision of masters projects:** encourage staff who have masters qualifications to retain their research skills. This can be done, for example, through collaborative arrangements with a local university. This might help identify research questions or provide masters student project supervision;
- **Clinical collaboration within multi-site trials:** encourage staff to seek opportunities

2.15

to engage with multi-centre trial work, in collaboration with medical, clinical and academic peers.

Employment of research posts: funding such posts is challenging, but possible if done in collaboration with medical colleagues. Use your professional body's sample post outlines as a template to build new job descriptions, and submit them to your local job evaluation panel to identify the banding.

How to disseminate research evidence

All the evidence in the world is of limited use if it is not disseminated and acted upon. This is dependent upon culture, the strength of the evidence and effective clinical leadership (Rycroft-Malone et al, 2004; Kitson, 2007). The following needs to be taken into account:
- **Culture:** a culture which is open and has a positive attitude to learning is one in which research evidence will be disseminated;
- **Evidence:** the strength of the evidence must be rigorously analysed and its significance to clinical practice assessed;
- **Leadership:** this is essential to demonstrate best practice, ensure that time is ring-fenced for CPD, allow effective learning to occur and monitor the implementation of that learning, until it has become part of the standard practice within the department.

How to sustain a capacity for research within a clinical environment

The competing demands within a clinical context represent a significant challenge. The needs of patients must come first, but the needs of patients will not be met in the long term without good governance arrangements and the evidence to support the practice. Realistic goals must be set for a sustainable level of research, and a pragmatic attitude to what research is and how it can be used to contribute to the operational and strategic needs of the therapy team.

How to sustain the research therapist

There are relatively few therapists employed in a clinical context who carry out research for the majority of their working week. These post holders are frequently in an isolated position.

As such it is recommended that:
- performance metrics are agreed and regularly assessed.
- mentorship is arranged.
- publications are encouraged.
- presentation at national and internal events is encouraged.
- effective support networking with other research professionals is provided.
- career development opportunities are investigated in collaboration with academic networks.

Conclusion

While being a research-oriented manager has many challenges, there are more than enough benefits to make it worthwhile to embrace research and use it to inform better patient care, better staff retention and better governance arrangements. In summary, the benefits are greater than the sum of the parts and if approached realistically, research can add value to the workings of therapy teams of the 21st century.

Reference list
- Borrill C et al. (2001) The Effectiveness of Health Care Teams in the National Health Service. Aston centre for Health Service Organisational Research, University of Aston.
- Cochrane A. (1976) Effectiveness and Efficiency. The Nuffield Trust. London
- Kitson A. (2007) What influences the use of research. Clinical Practice Nursing Research July/August Vol 56 no 4. Supplement: July/August 2007. Pages S1-S3
- Porter M, Teisberg E. (2006) Redefining Health Care: Creating Value-based Competition on Results. Harvard Business School Press, Boston.
- Rycroft-Malone J et al. (2004) An exploration of the factors that influence the implementation of evidence into practice. Journal of Clinical Nursing 13 (8), 913–924.
- West M et al. (2002). The link between management of employees and patient mortality in acute hospitals. International Journal of Human Resource Management, 13 (8), 1299-1310.

Further information
- Developing the Best Research Professionals. Report of the UKCRC Subcommittee for Nurses in Clinical Research. HMSO, London.

Glossary

Alpha the threshold probability value for statistical significance (for example an alpha of $p \leq 0.01$ means that an obtained p value at or below this level from a statistical test will denote statistical significance in respect of this test.

Alternative hypothesis an assumption that an effect or other statistical relationship exists in the population (for example that the population mean difference is greater or less than zero, that there is a non-zero positive or negative population correlation coefficient, or that the population odds ratio is other than unity). A two-tailed (two-sided) alternative hypothesis states that an effect exists but does not specify its direction (for example it predicts a non-zero mean difference that may be either positive or negative), whereas a one-tailed (one-sided) alternative hypothesis predicts a specific direction for an effect. If a statistical test rejects the null hypothesis, the alternative hypothesis is retained.

Central tendency measures of central tendency (such as the mode, median or mean) are averages, and indicate the 'typical' value in a set of data. A set of data can only have one mean or median value, but may have more than one mode.

Clinical guidelines published guidelines based on the best available evidence (usually randomised controlled trials). Designed to inform clinical practice.

Cognitive styles an individual's preferred way of perceiving/organising/using information to solve problems (for example one widely known cognitive style test is the Myers-Briggs Type Indicator).

Confidence interval a range of values on either side of the sample statistic, which we can be confident (for example 95 per cent confident in the case of a 95 per cent confidence interval) embraces the true population value. The confidence interval reflects the precision of the sample statistic as an estimate of the population parameter.

Continuous professional development (CPD) — CPD provides a framework for linking evidence with practice. Formally identifying sources of knowledge and evidence, critically reflecting on that evidence and describing how practice is influenced clarifies and formalises the link. CPD offers the opportunity to plan, act, record and review knowledge and its impact on practice.

Deduction — reasoning from the general to the specific or from a general premise to a particular situation.

Descriptive statistics — procedures that describe the statistical properties of a sample of observations.

Dispersion — measures of dispersion indicate the variability of a set of data measured at an ordinal, interval or ratio level, and include the range, interquartile range and standard deviation.

Epistemology — the branch of philosophy dealing with the ways in which knowledge of the world can be gained and assessed.

Ethical research — requires an approach that offers the greatest benefit to the greatest number of people, and minimises the potential for harm for participants, researchers and others.

Experiment — A research method used to establish cause-and-effect relationships between the independent and dependent variables by means of manipulation of variables, control and randomisation. A true experiment involves the random allocation of participants to experimental and control groups, manipulation of the independent

	variable, and the introduction of a control group (for comparison purposes). Participants are assessed before and after the manipulation of the independent variable in order to assess its effect on the dependent variable (the outcome).
Field notes	notes taken by researchers to record unstructured observations they make 'in the field' and their interpretation of those observations.
Focus group	an interview conducted with a small group of people to explore their ideas on a particular topic.
Hermeneutics	the study of meaning in actions, situations or objects.
Hypothesis	a tentative answer to a research question, expressed in the form of a prediction about the relationships between two or more variables.
Induction	reasoning from the specific to the general, where particular instances are observed and then combined into a larger theoretical statement.
Inferential statistics	procedures used on sample data that estimate, or test hypothesis relating to, a statistical property (parameter) of the population from which the sample of observations was drawn. Statistical tests and the use of confidence intervals are inferential procedures.
Interpretivism	the belief that researchers in their analysis of data must include the meanings that individuals give to events and behaviour.
Interview	a method of data collection involving an interviewer asking questions of another person (a respondent) either face-to-face or over the telephone. **Structured interview** the interviewer asks the respondents the same

questions using an interview schedule – a formal instrument that specifies the precise wording and ordering of all the questions to be asked of each respondent.
Semi- or unstructured interview
the researcher asks open-ended questions which give the respondent considerable freedom to talk freely on the topic and to influence the direction of the interview since there is no predetermined plan about the specific information to be gathered from those being interviewed.

Levels of measurement	a classification used to indicate the level of information within a variable, with the following categories: nominal, ordinal, interval, ratio. A nominal variable, for example, only contains information on category membership, whereas an ordinal variable contains in addition information on rank ordering.
Likert scale	a method used to measure attitudes, which involves respondents indicating their degree of agreement or disagreement with a series of statements. Scores are summed to give a composite measure of attitudes.
Methodology	the design and overall strategy for a research study, including the theoretical perspective held by the researcher.
Methods	the actual processes used to collect data (for example interviews, questionnaires).
Mixed methods	refers to research investigations that measure both quantitative data (for example how often a person breathes per minute) as well as collect and analyse qualitative data (for example interview or questionnaire about how the person feels when breathing).

Nonparametric statistics	statistical tests and other inferential procedures that make no – or minimal – assumptions about population parameters.
Null hypothesis	an assumption or prediction that an effect or other statistical relationship does not exist in the population (for examplethat the population mean difference is zero, that the population correlation coefficient is zero, or that the population odds ratio is unity). Statistical tests seek to reject the null hypothesis, in favour of the alternative hypothesis.
Observation	a method of data collection in which data are gathered through visual observations. **Structured observation** the researcher determines at the outset precisely what behaviours are to be observed and typically uses a standardised checklist to record the frequency with which those behaviours are observed over a specified time period. **Unstructured observation** the researcher uses direct observation to record behaviours as they occur, with no preconceived ideas of what will be seen; there is no predetermined plan about what will be observed.
Ontology	the branch of philosophy concerned with questions of what exists, or questions of being and reality.
Organisational effectiveness	how well an organisation is run, how effectively people are communicating and implementing their ideas and tasks.
Organisational exposure	when staff become noticed beyond their immediate line manager and colleagues through interacting with other departments and so on.
Paradigm	a set of beliefs, values and techniques, shared by the

	members of a given community, and constituting a 'worldview'.
Parametric statistics	statistical tests and other inferential procedures that make certain assumptions about population parameters, and whose appropriate use depends upon these assumptions being satisfied.
Peer mentee/mentor	a person on the same or a very similar level of knowledge and experience.
Phenomenology	an inductive, descriptive methodology developed from phenomenological philosophy for the purpose of describing experiences as they are lived by individuals.
Positivism	the belief that knowledge of the world can be detached from personal meaning and ethical evaluation.
Population parameter	the value of a certain statistical property of a population (for example population mean, population correlation coefficient, population proportion). The population parameter is fixed but unknown, and is therefore estimated by a sample statistic.
Probability value	most commonly, the p value from a statistical test, which indicates the probability that an effect of at least the observed magnitude would occur if the null hypothesis were true. A small p value therefore constitutes evidence against the null hypothesis, and if the p value lies at or below alpha, the null hypothesis is rejected.
Qualitative	refers to forms of data, data collection and data analysis that give priority to meaning over measurement.
Quantitative	refers to forms of data, data collection and data

analysis that give priority to measurement over meaning.

Quasi-experiment a type of experimental design where random assignment to groups is not employed for either ethical or practical reasons, but certain methods of control are employed and the independent variable is manipulated.

Research governance describes the regulations, principles and standards of good practice that exist to achieve, and continuously improve, research quality. Research governance is one of the core standards for healthcare organisations.

Research Governance Framework outlines the principles of good governance that apply to all research within the remit of the Secretary of State for Health, the mechanisms and monitoring arrangements that exist to ensure the standards are met.

Sample statistic the value of a certain statistical property of a sample (for example sample mean, sample correlation coefficient, sample proportion). The sample statistic is known because it can be measured, but being subject to random sampling error will vary from sample to sample from the same population. The sample statistic serves as an estimate of the corresponding population parameter.

Sampling the process of selecting a subgroup of a population to represent the entire population. There are several different types of sampling, including:
Probability sampling (random sampling)
this method gives each eligible element/unit an equal chance of being selected in the sample; random procedures are employed to select a sample using a sampling frame.
Purposive sampling
as its name would suggest, purposive sampling is about

selecting a particular sample on purpose, and is often used in qualitative research. The dimensions or factors according to which the sample is drawn up are analytically and theoretically linked to the research question(s) being addressed.

Systematic sampling
a probability sampling strategy involving the selection of participants randomly drawn from a population at fixed intervals (for example every 20th name from a sampling frame).

Cluster sampling
a probability sampling strategy involving successive sampling of units (or clusters); the units sample progress from larger ones to smaller ones (e.g. health authority/health board, trust, senior managers).

Convenience sampling (also referred to as accidental sampling)
a non-probability sampling strategy that uses the most easily accessible people (or objects) to participate in a study.

Quota sampling
a non-probability sampling strategy where the researcher identifies the various strata of a population and ensures that all these strata are proportionately represented within the sample to increase its representativeness.

Snowball sampling
a non-probability sampling strategy whereby referrals from earlier participants are used to gather the required number of participants.

Theoretical sampling
the selection of individuals within a naturalistic research study, based on emerging findings as the study progresses to ensure that key issues are adequately represented.

Statistical power   the probability that a statistical test will detect as significant an effect of a stated magnitude, where such

	an effect exists; for example the probability of rejecting a false null hypothesis. Sample size is normally the most important determinant of statistical power.
Statistical significance	a statistically significant finding is one that causes the corresponding null hypothesis to be rejected in a statistical test. The observed effect is taken to correspond to a 'real' effect in the population (rather than being simply the effect of a random sampling error from a population in which no such corresponding effect exists).
Triangulation	this term is used in a research context to describe the use of a variety of data sources or methods to examine a specific phenomenon either simultaneously or sequentially in order to produce a more accurate account of the phenomenon under investigation.
Type 1 error	the probability of a 'false positive' in a statistical test; that is the probability of rejecting a true null hypothesis. The Type 1 error rate is alpha, the chosen threshold for statistical significance.
Type 2 error	the probability of a 'false negative' in a statistical test; that is the probability of failing to reject a false null hypothesis. The Type 2 error rate is beta, and is the complement of statistical power (that is if beta is 0.10, power is 0.90).
Variables	qualities or properties of persons, things or situations that change or can take different values in different cases and are manipulated or measured in research.

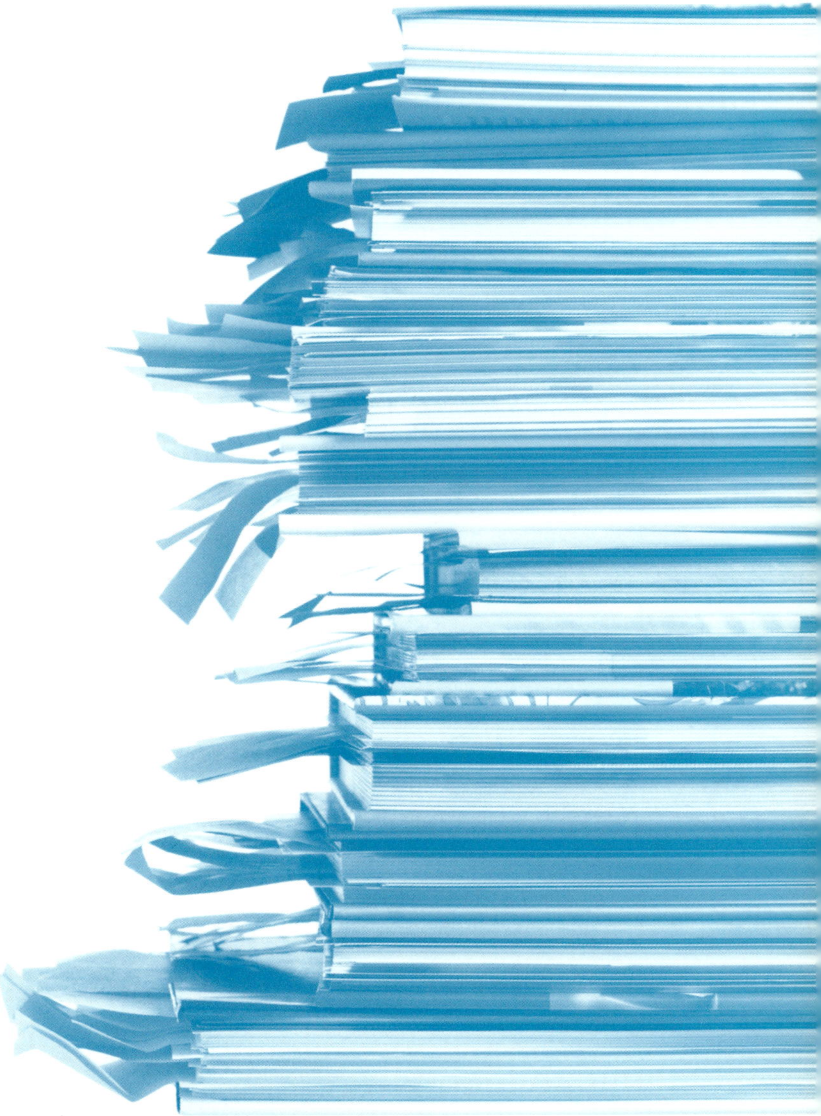

Brief biographies of contributors

Rhoda Allison
Rhoda Allison is Consultant Therapist for Stroke at Devon PCT and an Honorary Research Fellow at the Primary Care Department of the Peninsula Medical School. She combines a clinical role as lead for Stroke Rehabilitation and Spasticity management, with research. She has a particular interest in health promotion and user involvement, and has been involved in both quantitative and qualitative research studies. She is currently involved in conducting an action research project looking at secondary prevention advice for people after stroke. She was previously a member of the CSP's Research and Clinical Effectiveness Committee, and the Clinical Guidelines Endorsement Panel, and is currently the invited expert for physiotherapy for the Clinical Guidelines Development Group for the NICE guideline for Acute Stroke and TIA.

David Baxter
David Baxter is Professor and Dean of the School of Physiotherapy, University of Otago, New Zealand. He completed an honours degree in physiotherapy in 1987, and his doctorate (DPhil) in 1991 at the University of Ulster, where he subsequently held various positions including Head of Research Graduate School and Head of School of Rehabilitation Sciences before moving to Otago in 2005. David's areas of teaching interest include electrophysical agents, research methods, and pain management. His research interests are varied and include the non-pharmacological management of musculoskeletal pain (particularly low back pain), laser therapy, and complementary and alternative medicine. During his career he has achieved recognition for his research on physiotherapy and rehabilitation, as part of which he has authored or edited two books, four book chapters, and 100 full papers in peer-reviewed scientific and clinical journals. He is Editor-in-Chief of Physical Therapy Reviews, the only review journal in the field, and is an editorial board member for several other international journals. David has a particular interest in graduate research training, and has supervised 37 PhDs to successful completion. He was previously a member of the UK Council for Graduate Education's Executive Council, and acted as convenor for the Council's Working Group on Research Training in the Healthcare Professions, which reported in 2003.

Anne Bruton
After working clinically as a specialist respiratory physiotherapist, Anne Bruton undertook a second degree in Biological Anthropology at the University of Cambridge, acquiring First Class honours. Anne joined the School of Health Professions and Rehabilitation Sciences (SHPRS), University of Southampton in 1994 as a Lecturer in Physiotherapy and her health research career began in 1997 when she was awarded a Department of Health Research Studentship to undertake a full-time PhD. Her thesis was entitled

'The evaluation and application of a new measure of inspiratory muscle function'. Subsequently she was awarded a Department of Health Postdoctoral Research Fellowship (2003–6) for a research programme entitled 'Investigations into the physiological basis for Buteyko breathing training and its effectiveness as complementary therapy for patients with asthma'. She is currently Reader in Respiratory Rehabilitation at the University of Southampton and Deputy Director of Research for SHPRS. She is Chair of the CSP Research & Clinical Effectiveness Group and sits on several other national respiratory and research committees.

Mindy Cairns
Mindy is Senior Lecturer and Research Lead for Physiotherapy at the University of Hertfordshire. She qualified in 1991 as a physiotherapist from Guy's Hospital and initially worked at St Bartholomew's Hospital, London. After specialising in neuromusculoskeletal physiotherapy, she undertook a full-time MSc (Manipulative Therapy) at Coventry University and gained MACP membership in 1997. Following this, she took a clinical research post at the Royal Orthopaedic Hospital, Birmingham and completed her PhD in 2002. She has presented and published her research work nationally and internationally and continues to be involved in clinical research. Mindy has taught extensively as a visiting lecturer on MSc courses and been involved in developing masters level modules within the MSc neuromusculoskeletal framework at UH. Her clinical and research interests include spinal stability in the management of low back pain, outcome measures and clinically based therapy research. She has been Research Officer for the MACP since 2002.

Elizabeth Cousins
Elizabeth Cousins qualified as a physiotherapist in 1993 from the Manchester Royal Infirmary School of Physiotherapy. Since graduating, she has worked in various hospitals in Manchester and the West Midlands, specialising in neurological rehabilitation. She is currently undertaking a PhD full-time at the University of Keele, where she is researching aspects of the recovery of grip post stroke.

Janet Deane
Janet qualified with an honours degree in physiotherapy from King's College, London in 2001. Since qualifying Janet has worked at Guy's and St Thomas' hospital. As a Senior Physiotherapist she contributed to various specialist areas of musculoskeletal care as well as the undergraduate physiotherapy teaching programme at King's College London. In 2006, Janet completed an MSc in Advanced Musculoskeletal Rehabilitation at University

College London and qualified as a member of the Manipulative Association of Chartered Physiotherapists. During this time she developed a specialist interest in hypermobility and injuries related to the performing arts and worked with the British Association of Performing Arts Medicine (BAPAM). Janet currently works in the private sector and as a research physiotherapist at Imperial College London.

Krysia Dziedzic

Krysia Dziedzic qualified as a physiotherapist at Manchester Royal Infirmary (1982). She began her clinical career at Withington (Manchester), later moving to Sevenoaks and then to the Medway Hospitals (Kent) specialising in rheumatology and hand therapy. She then moved to the Staffordshire Rheumatology Centre, Stoke on Trent, to a rheumatology research post. She completed a PhD at Keele University (1997) and became a Senior Research Fellow and West Midlands Physiotherapy Clinical Trialist in the Primary Care Musculoskeletal Research Centre (Keele University). She was appointed ARC Senior Lecturer in Physiotherapy. Her research portfolio includes applied clinical studies in osteoarthritis. She has held a number of positions related to Rheumatology including: President British Health Professionals in Rheumatology (2002–2004) Steering Committee member National Electronic Library for Health/Musculoskeletal branch (2003-2005), Arthritis and Musculoskeletal Alliance (ARMA) coordinator Osteoarthritis Standards of Care (2002–2005). Participated in two EULAR guidelines for the management and diagnosis of hand osteoarthritis (2005–2007). Guideline Development Group Member NICE Osteoarthritis guidelines (2006–2008).Currently she is a member of the ARC Research and Academic Capacity Committee

Caroline Ellis-Hill

Caroline Ellis-Hill is currently a Senior Lecturer at the School of Health Professions and Rehabilitation Sciences, University of Southampton. She has been working in the field of qualitative research since 1994 when she started her PhD entitled 'New world, new rules: life narratives and changes in self concept in the first year after stroke' which was funded by a Department of Health Research Studentship, awarded in 1998. She has worked on several research studies involving qualitative research using methodologies such as narrative approaches, focus groups, grounded theory and Delphi techniques in areas related to long-term conditions such as Parkinson's disease, stroke and spinal cord injury.

Claudia Fellmer

Claudia Fellmer obtained her first academic degree in Germany and then moved to Southampton, UK to complete a PhD in Cultural and Film Studies, while teaching in the Modern Languages Department. In 2004, she joined the School of Health Professions and Rehabilitation Sciences (since July 2008 School of Health Sciences) at the University of Southampton as Research Manager. Her day-to-day business involved the administration of research related tasks, such as ethics committees, grant application preparations, preparing reports on the school's research profile, supporting the running of conferences and looking after the student life cycle for the doctorate programmes. In 2007 she obtained an MBA; her dissertation investigated research mentoring in an academic environment. While this book was being completed she took up a post with Southampton University Hospitals NHS trust working as Research Governance and Quality Assurance Manager.

Laura Finucane

Laura qualified as a physiotherapist in 1996 from Brunel University. In 2003 she completed her MSc in Manipulative Physiotherapy at Brighton University. She completed her dissertation on cardiovascular fitness and low back pain. Since 2006 she has worked as a Consultant Musculoskeletal Physiotherapist specialising in spinal conditions and is the clinical lead for three musculoskeletal interface services. As a visiting fellow of the University of Brighton she examines Masters students and is a mentor to students undertaking MACP placements. As a member of the Professional Executive Committee for Surrey PCT she is a clinical champion for health improvement. She is also involved in redesigning Orthopaedic services across the PCT. Laura is a member of the Manipulation Association of Chartered Physiotherapist (MACP) executive committee where she is the International Federation of Manual Therapists (IFOMT) member organisation delegate. She is involved in the South East Thames musculoskeletal research group which helps to facilitate research locally. She is a reviewer for Manual Therapy Journal.

Nadine Foster

One of the senior academic team in the Clinical Trials Unit of the Arthritis Research Campaign National Primary Care Centre at Keele University, Nadine is a physiotherapist whose research activity is focused on musculoskeletal healthcare. Her research includes clinical trials in the field of low back pain and knee pain, with specific interests in evidence-based practice in primary care, patients' and practitioners' attitudes about pain and the process of care for patients. Her portfolio of research includes studies of the effectiveness of interventions across the spectrum of physiotherapists, general practitioners, osteopaths and chiropractors. With a track record of more than £10 million research funding and 50 full paper publications, she has supervised 12 MSc/MMedSci and six PhD students to completion. She lectures on the MSc Neuromusculoskeletal Healthcare programme and MSc Pain Sciences and Management programmes at Keele

University. Previously she was the research representative on the CSP's governing council and her current post is funded through a primary care career scientist award from the National Insitute of Health Research (NIHR), to deliver a programme of research on musculoskeletal problems.

Stuart Fraser
Stuart graduated from the University of Southampton in 1999 with a BSc in Physiotherapy. He initially worked in Worthing Hospital before moving to Southampton University Hospitals trust, where he currently works as a senior clinician in the Wessex Neurological Centre, a regional neurological and neurosurgical unit. He has lectured on BSc and MSc physiotherapy courses and presented research on Cauda Equina Syndrome at the Society for Back Pain Research and at the 2007 World Confederation for Physical Therapy conference in Vancouver. Stuart's current research interests are in red flags and Cauda Equina Syndrome.

Adam Garrow
After working as a full-time podiatrist in the NHS for eight years, Dr Garrow embarked on his research career on completion of an MSc in Medical Research Methods at Loughborough of Technology. He was awarded his PhD in Epidemiology at the Arthritis Research Campaign (ARC) Epidemiology Research Unit at the University of Manchester. In 2002 he moved from musculoskeletal disease to diabetes and worked for 5 years as a Research Fellow at the Manchester Diabetes Centre, specialising on lower limb diabetic complications, before taking up his current research position at the University of Salford. Dr Garrow currently works for Health RDS NoW and part of his role is to support NHS researchers who would like to submit research grant and research fellowship applications. He is also developing an interest in Complementary and Alternative Medicine (CAM) and has recently secured NIHR funding to carry out CAM randomised controlled trials in diabetes and cancer.

Helen Hampson
Helen Hampson is a Research & Development Officer at the College of Occupational Therapists. Helen joined the college in 2006 to take a lead role in ensuring the activities of the college and its business groups fulfill research governance requirements, and provide an expert resource on research governance for the membership. In her previous role at St Bartholomew's School of Nursing & Midwifery, City University, Helen led the school's research administration office, and successfully completed an MSc in Social Research Methods.

Michele Harms
Michele Harms is the Editor in Chief of Physiotherapy Journal. She is a member of the Council of Science Editors and a Fellow of the Royal Statistical Society. She acts as a reviewer for a number of other journals including the British Medical Journal, Rheumatology, Clinical Biomechanics and Manual Therapy Journal. She completed an MSc in Ergonomics at Loughborough University and went on to study for her PhD with the University of London. Her areas of research interest have been varied and included orthopaedics, cardiac rehabilitation and musculoskeletal medicine. She is particularly interested in research design and statistics.

Bernadette Henderson
Bernadette Henderson is currently practising as an Advanced Clinical Practitioner in Cardiorespiratory Physiotherapy, and is the Clinical Governance Lead for Therapies and Dietetics, at Barnet and Chase Farm Hospitals NHS Trust. Bernadette completed her MSc in Cardiorespiratory Physiotherapy (Distinction) at University College London in 1997 and then led the Cardiorespiratory MSc programme at UCL from 1999–2004. Bernadette is currently in the fourth year of her professional doctorate at Brighton University, her research study is entitled 'Experienced cardiorespiratory physiotherapists' understandings of their interactive behaviour with chronically breathless patients.'

Rupert Kerrell
Rupert Kerrell graduated from Brunel University College in 1998. He returned there in 2000 to study part-time for his MSc in Neurorehabilitation which he successfully completed in 2003. During this time he worked for St. George's Hospital NHS trust mainly in the neurology department completing rotations in neurology, neurosurgery, neurorehabilitation and acute stroke. He continued to work as a Senior I in elderly rehabilitation and acute geriatrics before leaving the NHS in 2005 to work as a research assistant. The research project (which lasted 2 1/2 years) evaluated a number of new courses designed to train pre-registration allied health professionals (occupational therapists, physiotherapists, diagnostic and therapeutic radiographers) at two London universities. Since October 2007 he has been working as a Senior Lecturer in Occupational Therapy in the Department of Allied Health Professions at Canterbury Christ Church University.

Jeremy Lewis
Jeremy Lewis is research lead for the Therapy Department at Chelsea and Westminster Hospital, London. He is also a consultant physiotherapist at St George's Hospital in London and is a visiting reader at St George's, University of London. Jeremy has lead

clinical research in the areas of musculoskeletal disease, gerontology, cardio-respiratory physiotherapy, patients with burns injuries, hand therapy and hypermobility syndromes. His main area of research interest is rotator cuff pathology and shoulder pain. He is currently supervising a number of PhD and MSc students and is a member of the senior researchers forum at the Chartered Society of Physiotherapy.

Philippa Lyon

Philippa Lyon was Research Officer to the National Physiotherapy Research Network from 2005–2008, promoting the network and coordinating and supporting the 20 regional research hubs. Prior to this she had a number of years' experience working in university research support and management, and a parallel career in research and teaching in her own field of English Literature. She wrote a number of reports and articles on research capacity building in the therapy professions while in her post as NPRN Research Officer.

Brona McDowell

Brona McDowell joined the Gait Analysis Service at Musgrave Park Hospital in 1998 and currently works as a Clinical Specialist. As well as undertaking a clinical role within the laboratory, she has been involved in several research projects that have focused on children with myelomeningocele and cerebral palsy (CP). A randomised placebo-controlled trial assessing the efficacy of electrical stimulation for strengthening muscle in children with CP was completed in 2003 and current research focuses on population studies of the (i) mild to moderately and (ii) severely involved children with this condition. Within these studies, orthopaedic problems, gait (as applicable), functional ability, participation and service provision have been key areas of focus. She has acheived 25 full paper publications, has supervised one MPhil and two PhD students through to completion of their work, and sits on the editorial board of the journals *Gait and Posture* and *Physical and Occupational Therapy in Pediatric Research*.

Sue Mawson

Sue Mawson is Professor of Rehabilitation in the Centre for Health and Social Care Research. She joined the university in November 1991 to undertake a funded doctorate in the area of stroke rehabilitation. This research completed in 1997, was jointly funded by the Sheffield Teaching Hospitals NHS trust. Dr. Mawson qualified as a physiotherapist working predominantly in adult and child neurological rehabilitation. She is Research Lead for the Professional Services Directorate at Sheffield Teaching Hospitals representing the AHPs at both a local and national level. Prof Mawson's research focuses on improving the quality of life of people with neurological problems, particularly through exploration of the effectiveness of rehabilitative interventions. Her particular area of interest has been in the quantification of patient-centred goals working with the TELER methods of outcome measurements to developing valid and reliable ways of demonstrating efficient and effective intervention strategies. Prof Mawson currently has four full-time and two part-time PhD students working on neurological, musculoskeletal and respiratory rehabilitation and falls prevention. Her research work, funded predominantly through the Engineering and Physical Science Research Council, has capitalised on new innovations in sensor and digital technologies and involves interdisciplinary work, integrating clinical rehabilitation researchers with engineering, design, mecatronics, informatics and digital media specialists. This work has been driven by the needs of people with long-term conditions, identifying new ways of motivating and supporting them through the self-management of rehabilitation goals using technology innovations. The SMART 1 project, which commenced in 2003, was awarded £670K funding and has now led to a formal collaboration with Philips electronics, Aachen, Germany, and two further projects. 'Target', to further develop the SMART prototypes in preparation for clinical testing and SMART 2 extending the concept of self-management in stroke rehabilitation to self-management of Chronic Pain interventions and Chronic Heart Failure care (EPSRC £2.9 million).

Suzanne McDonough

Suzanne McDonough is Professor of Health and Rehabilitation at the University of Ulster, Northern Ireland. She is a physiotherapist by background and she was awarded her PhD in the area of neurophysiology in 1995 and a higher diploma in healthcare (acupuncture) in 2002. She has published widely in her areas of expertise and has published several chapters on electrotherapy in key textbooks for example *Electrotherapy: Evidence Based Practice* (2008), and *Animal Physiotherapy. Assessment, Treatment and Rehabilitation of Animals* (2007). She has also recently published a chapter on acupuncture in *Complementary Therapies for Physical Therapy. A Clinical Decision Making Approach* published by Elsevier in 2008. She has obtained funding from a variety of prestigious external agencies and is currently completing several clinical trials on musculoskeletal pain, one of which is investigating the effects of acupuncture as an adjunct to an exercise programme in people with low back pain. Her research interests include electrotherapy/acupuncture and developing technologies used for musculoskeletal and neurological rehabilitation. She has played a key role in helping to develop research in physiotherapy. She teaches clinical research techniques at undergraduate and postgraduate level and has supervised 14 PhD students to completion. She is part of the research group at the University of Ulster who were
top rated for physiotherapy research in the last two research assessment exercises (1996 and 2001).

Ann Moore

Ann qualified as a physiotherapist from Coventry School of Physiotherapy in 1973 and worked clinically until 1977. She then undertook a teaching course at Wolverhampton Polytechnic and specialised in musculoskeletal physiotherapy, becoming a member of the MACP in 1979. In 1980 she took up a teaching/research post at Coventry Polytechnic and later registered for a PhD programme on exercise and low back pain. She completed her PhD in 1989 and moved to the University of Brighton in 1991
where she is now Director of the Clinical Research Centre for Health Professions and Professor of Physiotherapy. She has more than 100 peer review publications and is a frequently invited keynote speaker at national and international conferences. Ann has been an active researcher since 1980 with interests in musculoskeletal physiotherapy, patients' experiences, standardised data collection, as well as pedagogic research.
She has supervised a number of PhD students to completion. Ann is currently Chair of the National Physiotherapy Research Network Core Executive and Executive Editor of Manual *Therapy Journal*.

Gail Mountain

Professor Gail Mountain is an academic occupational therapist with over 13 years experience as a practitioner and manager in services for older people and people with mental health problems. She embarked upon a research career in 1987, working at the University of Leeds. During this time Gail also obtained an MPhil in social psychology. She then moved to the University of York. A three-year return to the health service in 1991 was followed by employment as a researcher at the Nuffield Institute for Health, University of Leeds where she also obtained her doctorate. In 1998, Gail was employed as the first Research and Development officer at the College of Occupational Therapists, UK. In 2001 she moved to Sheffield Hallam University to lead research across nursing, allied health and social work. She was Director of the Centre for Health and Social Care Research at Sheffield Hallam University from 2003 to the beginning of 2008, and is now the Director of the Smart Consortium, funded by the Engineering and Physical Sciences Research Council.

Di Newham

Di Newham (PhD FCSP) is currently Director of the multidisciplinary Division of Applied Biomedical Research at King's College London (KCL). Prior to that she was Head of the Academic Department of Physiotherapy at KCL from 1989–1993. That post followed more than ten years working in full-time research in the Departments of Medicine and Physiology at University College London. After qualification as a physiotherapist she specialised in musculoskeletal and neurological physiotherapy. She has published more than 100 original research papers and been awarded research funding totalling in excess of £2m. She has been a member of research and strategic committees of a number of medical research charities and is part of the Core Executive of the NPRN. Her research interests focus on skeletal muscle function, ageing and rehabilitation.

Fiona Ottewell
As Head of Physiotherapy Gateshead Health NHS Foundation trust Fiona ensures the operational management and clinical governance of the department (113 WTE). She has led processes for Quality Improvement and Patient Experience within the Therapies Directorate. She has also been the NHS EMPLOYERS AHP/HCS Policy Board representative and represented NHS Employers on the Skills for Health Allied Health Professions Career Framework Strategy Group. In addition Fiona sat on the new working party for the modernisation of healthcare professionals. She has also been a Healthcare Commission Clinical Advisor, undertaken one review of a PCT for CHI in 2003–2004 and been a clinical advisor on several cases. She represents the trust at a local, regional and national level. One of the recent highlights in her career was to recruit a research physiotherapist in partnership with her trust's orthopaedic department and the local university.

Lorna Paul
Lorna Paul (PhD MPhil BSc) worked as a lecturer in physiotherapy at Glasgow Caledonian University for more than 13 years Lorna has recently taken up the post of Reader within Nursing and Health Care at the University of Glasgow. Her research interests include the measurement of function, multiple sclerosis, diabetes and chronic fatigue syndrome. She is one of the two coordinators of the West of Scotland hub of the National Physiotherapy Research Network and is a member of the Research and Clinical Effectiveness Committee of the Chartered Society of Physiotherapy.

Andrea Peace
Andrea Peace (BA, MA, MCLIP) is Head of Professional Policy and Information at the Chartered Society of Physiotherapy. Andrea is a chartered library and information professional and has worked in the health information field for the last 13 years, previously in the university sector as a faculty librarian/site manager, and for the last six years at the Chartered Society of Physiotherapy where she manages the library and information service. Andrea is a member of the executive committee for the Consortium of Health Independent Libraries in London (CHILL) which exists to provide the independent health libraries in the London area with opportunities to improve their services through mutual communication and cooperation.

Nikki Petty

Nikki Petty qualified as a chartered physiotherapist from Newcastle Polytechnic in 1979. She completed a graduate diploma in Manipulative Therapy in Melbourne Australia and later completed a research dissertation to gain an MSc from Coventry University. She is currently Principal Lecturer at the School of Health Professions, University of Brighton. She teaches neuromusculoskeletal physiotherapy at undergraduate and postgraduate level and is course leader for the MSc Neuromusculoskeletal Physiotherapy. She has written two successful textbooks on neuromusculoskeletal examination and assessment, and neuromusculoskeletal treatment and management. She has a number of research publications mostly related to the application of spinal accessory movements within the field of neuromusculoskeletal physiotherapy. She is on the international advisory board of *Manual Therapy*, an international journal of musculoskeletal therapy and has served on the advisory board of the *Journal of Manual and Manipulative Therapy*. She acts as a reviewer for both peer reviewed journals. She has presented widely at conferences in the UK and abroad, with several as an invited speaker. She is currently a member of the MACP Executive Committee, and Chair and founder member of the MACP Committee for Education and Approval. At the time of press, she is in the final stages of completing her Professional Doctorate in Physiotherapy at the University of Brighton. The research study is within her professional practice as an educator and is focused on the learning transition of neuromusculoskeletal physiotherapists towards criticality of practice knowledge.

Gabrielle Rankin

Gabrielle Rankin works three days as a research adviser at the CSP and two days in clinical practice. As a research adviser, her main roles are to support and advise members on all aspects of research, to promote physiotherapy research and to influence relevant health research policy. Gabrielle works in close collaboration with the NPRN and also with the other allied health professions. She sits on the Core Executive of the NRPN and on the Research Forum for Allied Health Professions. Clinical and research interests are in the field of musculoskeletal physiotherapy. Specific areas of interest that she has published in are rehabilitative ultrasound imaging which was the topic of her PhD, muscle rehabilitation, ergonomics and the classification and management of low back pain. Gabrielle is an associate editor of *Physiotherapy* and a member of the International Advisory Board of *Manual Therapy* Journal.

Lisa Roberts

Lisa Roberts trained at St Thomas' Hospital, London, and has worked at Southampton university since 1989. She is a senior lecturer at the University of Southampton and superintendent physiotherapist at Southampton University Hospitals trust, working in the musculoskeletal outpatient department. Her PhD was in control issues and low back pain and her current research interests are back pain, communication, clinical reasoning, red flags, self-report outcome measures and ethical reasoning. Lisa is a trustee and member of the Research Committee of BackCare (formerly the National Back Pain Association); vice-chair of the Southampton Branch of BackCare, secretary for the Society for Back Pain Research; and provides a link with clinicians in the Southampton Hub of the National Physiotherapy Research Network.

Julius Sim

Julius Sim (BA MSc(Soc) MSc(Stat) PhD) is Professor of Health Care Research at Keele University, where he teaches statistics and research methods to postgraduate students. He is currently involved in research in musculoskeletal pain, social gerontology and applied ethics. Julius is a member of the Core Executive of the National Physiotherapy Research Network.

Sally Singh

Professor Sally Singh is based at Coventry University, in the School of Physiotherapy (Faculty of Health and Life Sciences) and at the University Hospitals of Leicester NHS Trust. She was awarded her PhD in 1993 and since that time has been involved in the development of Pulmonary and Cardiac Rehabilitation Services. Her research interests initially focused on the development of robust outcome measures to evaluate these complex interventions. More recently research activity has focused upon service delivery models and the application of exercise therapy in the acute setting. The physiological and metabolic response to exercise in patients with chronic cardio-respiratory disease is also of interest to the research group and some recent publications have explored this. She is an editor of a journal and associate editor of '*Physiotherapy*'. She is Vice Chair of the Research and Clinical Effectiveness Committee for the Chartered Society of Physiotherapy. She has just completed a term as Chair of the American Thoracic Society Pulmonary Rehabilitation Group and is the incoming Chair of the European Respiratory Society Pulmonary Rehabilitation Group.

Graham Stew

Graham Stew is a Principal Lecturer in the School of Health Professions at the University of Brighton, and also Programme Leader for the Professional Doctorate in Health and Social Care. He has a background in mental health nursing and education, and enjoys teaching most aspects of the research process. Having gained general and mental health nursing qualifications in 1974, and worked within therapeutic communities in London and Cambridge, he moved into nurse education in 1982 and university teaching in 1988, gaining his DPhil in education in 1994. Graham's current academic and research interests include: practitioner research methodologies; reflective practice; interprofessional education and the teaching of mindfulness meditation.

Maria Stokes

Professor Maria Stokes (PhD MCSP) began a career in research two years after qualifying as a physiotherapist, studying for a PhD (CNAA) in Neuromuscular Physiology at the Nuffield Department of Orthopaedic Surgery and Department of Zoology at the University of Oxford. As a postdoctoral research fellow in Clinical Physiology at the Department of Medicine, University of Liverpool, she investigated the physiological mechanisms of muscle weakness and fatigue. She spent four years as a senior lecturer in the Department of Physiotherapy, University of Queensland, Australia, focusing more on developing investigative techniques, specifically ultrasound imaging of muscle and mechanomyography (muscle sounds). She then returned to England as Director of Research & Development at the Royal Hospital for Neurodisability, Putney, London, where she continued her previous research interests, which extended to brain-computer interfacing (BCI) technology. Maria took up her current post in 2004 as Professor in Neuromuscular Rehabilitation and Director of Research in the School of Health Professions and Rehabilitation Sciences at the University of Southampton. Her research focuses on physiological mechanisms of muscle function in healthy populations and people with musculoskeletal disorders, and neurological conditions. She leads the School's Musculoskeletal Research Theme, but much of her research activity overlaps with the Neurorehabilitation Theme. Maria has published her research widely in the scientific literature and has also published four books. Maria is a member of the Core Executive of the National Physiotherapy Research Network.

Elizabeth White

Elizabeth completed her PhD in Social Policy in 1997, and has been Head of Research and Development at the College of Occupational Therapists since 2003. Her remit includes the strategic promotion of occupational therapy R&D, development of the United Kingdom Occupational Therapy Research Foundation and facilitating research activity among the college's membership. She represents the profession on the NICE Partners' Council, the SDO Programme Board, is a member of the Research Forum for Allied Health Professions and represents the RFAHP on the National Physiotherapy Research Network Core executive.